ESSENTIAL
CHAKRA
YOGA

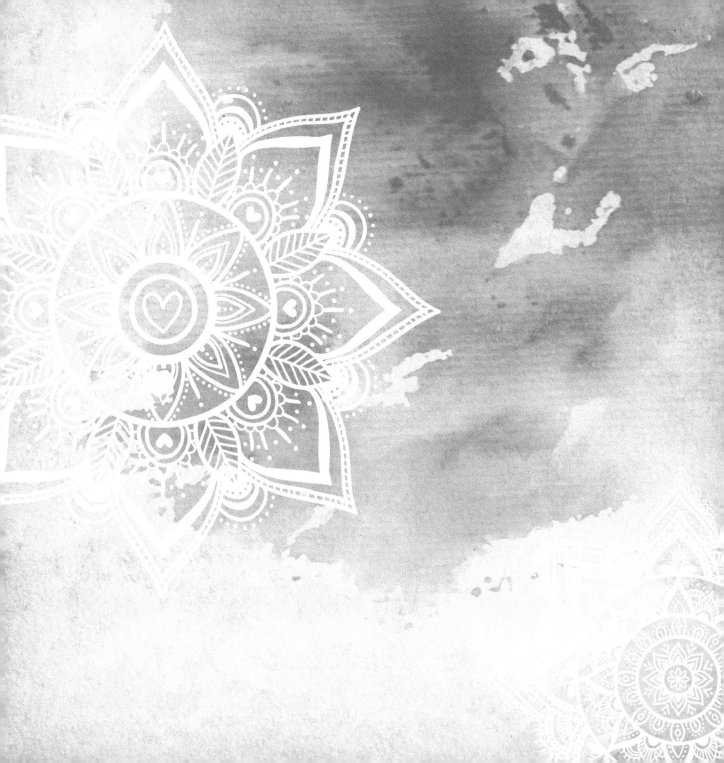

ESSENTIAL
CHAKRA YOGA

POSES TO BALANCE, HEAL, AND ENERGIZE THE BODY AND MIND

CHRISTINA D'ARRIGO

Illustrations by Amanda León

ROCKRIDGE PRESS

Interior Designer: Michael Patti
Cover Designer: Julie Gueraseva
Art Producer: Hillary Frileck
Editor: Sean Newcott
Production Editor: Rachel Taenzler

Illustrations © 2019 Amanda León

Author photo courtesy of © Allison Armfield

ISBN: Print 978-1-64611-450-4 | eBook 978-1-64611-451-1

R1

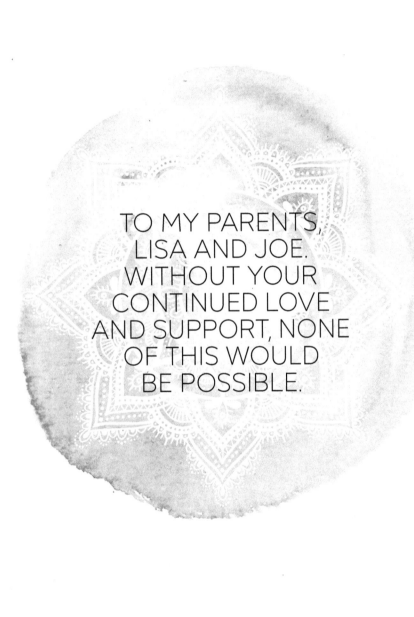

TO MY PARENTS,
LISA AND JOE.
WITHOUT YOUR
CONTINUED LOVE
AND SUPPORT, NONE
OF THIS WOULD
BE POSSIBLE.

CONTENTS

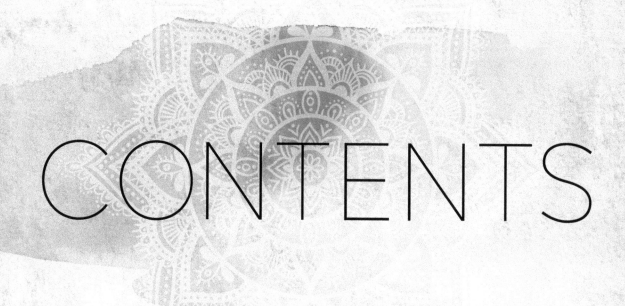

INTRODUCTION x

PART 1: CONNECTING THE MIND AND BODY 1

CHAPTER 1
the harmony of chakra and yoga 2

CHAPTER 2
discovering the chakras 9

CHAPTER 3
beginning your chakra yoga practice 20

PART 2: HEALING THROUGH CHAKRA YOGA 31

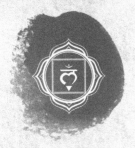

CHAPTER 4

root chakra 32

Siddhasana:
Accomplished Pose 33

Anjaneyasana: Low Lunge
(Variation with the Knee Down) 34

Baddha Konasana: Bound-Angle
Pose 35

Ananda Balasana:
Happy Baby Pose 36

Prasarita Padottanasana I:
Wide-Legged Forward Bend 37

Upavistha Konasana:
Wide-Angle Pose 38

Malasana: Garland Pose 39

Kapotasana: Pigeon Pose 40

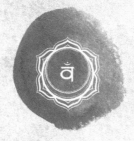

CHAPTER 5

sacral chakra 41

Paschimottanasana:
Seated Forward Bend 42

Janu Sirsasana:
Head-to-Knee Forward Bend 43

Setu Bandha Sarvangasana:
Bridge Pose 44

Adho Mukha Svanasana:
Downward-Facing Dog Pose 45

Navasana: Boat Pose 46

Ashta Chandrasana:
High Lunge 47

Virabhadrasana II:
Warrior II Pose 48

Utkata Konasana:
Goddess Pose 49

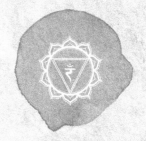

CHAPTER 6

solar plexus chakra 50

Marjaryasana: Cat Pose 51

Bitilasana: Cow Pose 52

Ardha Matsyendrasana:
Half Lord of the Fishes Pose 53

Utthita Trikonasana:
Extended Triangle Pose 54

Bhujangasana: Cobra Pose 55

Urdhva Mukha Svanasana:
Upward-Facing Dog Pose 56

Dhanurasana: Bow Pose 57

Natarajasana: Dancer Pose 58

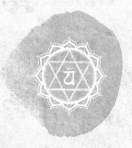

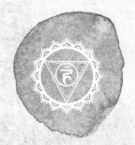

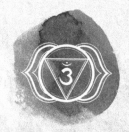

CHAPTER 7

heart chakra 59

Tadasana: Mountain Pose
(Variation with Hands Clasped) 60

Ardha Bhujangasana:
Low Cobra Pose 61

Salamba Bhujangasana: Sphinx or
Supported Cobra Pose 62

Anahatasana:
Melting Heart Pose 63

Camatkarasana: Wild Thing 64

Matsyasana: Fish Pose 65

Ustrasana: Camel Pose 66

Urdhva Dhanurasana:
Upward-Facing Bow or
Wheel Pose 67

CHAPTER 8

throat chakra 69

Assisted Neck Stretches in
Sukhasana: Easy Pose 70

Neck Rolls in Sukhasana:
Easy Pose 72

Sukhasana with Jalandhara
Bandha: Easy Pose with
Chin Lock 73

Salamba Matsyasana:
Supported Fish Pose 74

Ashtangasana:
Knees, Chest, Chin Pose 75

Uttanasana:
Standing Forward Bend 76

Halasana: Plow Pose 77

Salamba Sarvangasana:
Supported Shoulder Stand 78

CHAPTER 9

third-eye chakra 79

Balasana: Child's Pose 80

Prone Savasana:
Prone Corpse Pose 81

Kumbhakasana: Plank Pose 82

Chaturanga Dandasana:
Four-Limbed Staff Pose 83

Viparita Karani:
Legs Up the Wall Pose 84

Baddha Konasana Variation:
Butterfly Pose 85

Gomukhasana: Cow Face Pose 87

Adho Mukha Vrksasana:
Handstand 89

CHAPTER 10

crown chakra 91

Tadasana: Mountain Pose 92

Savasana: Corpse Pose 93

Vrksasana: Tree Pose 94

Anjaneyasana Variation: Crescent Lunge with Arms Up 95

Vasisthasana: Side Plank Pose 96

Utthita Parsvakonasana: Extended Side-Angle Pose 97

Ardha Chandrasana: Half-Moon Pose 98

Salamba Sirsasana: Supported Headstand 99

CHAPTER 11

healing multiple chakras 101

Activating and Grounding the Midsection 102

Drawing Attention and Focus to the Upper Chakras 105

Paying Attention to the Extremities 108

Building a Strong Foundation 111

CHAPTER 12

healing your inner self 116

Strength Building for the Whole Body 117

Energizing the Full Body 121

Calming and Relaxing the Mind and Body 126

Keeping the Full Body Grounded and Centered 129

INDEX 132

INTRODUCTION

HELLO! WELCOME TO the world of chakra yoga! I am so happy that you found this book and are on your way to discovering how much healing you can achieve through practicing yoga and learning more about the chakras.

I began my yoga journey in a yoga for dancers class, which I was required to take while studying for my bachelor's degree in dance. About six years later, after practicing yoga recreationally at gyms and in yoga studios, I decided I wanted to dive deeper into yoga and get my teacher-training certification. I completed the first 200 hours of my yoga-teacher training in one month, and it completely changed my life. About a year later, I added 300 additional hours to that certification, and I have been teaching and practicing yoga ever since.

I came to learn more about the chakras while trying to solve my own issues with generalized anxiety disorder. I wanted to see if energy was blocked in certain areas of my body and whether there were specific poses I should be doing more often to release that energy and achieve less anxiety in my life. Through this research, I became completely fascinated with the chakra system. As I reached a deeper understanding about the chakras, I began to incorporate chakra balancing into my personal yoga practice.

For instance, I discovered that during a panic attack, I held a lot of tension in my heart chakra. Once I knew that, when I had a panic attack or felt one coming on, I focused my energy and did particular yoga poses or sequences to alleviate some of the tightness and discomfort I was experiencing in that area. I also discovered other areas that needed attention, and with my understanding of the chakras, I am now able to continually work toward finding balance and harmony throughout my body.

A chakra yoga practice is very rewarding, and you are able to get a lot more out of your yoga practice when you pay close attention to the chakras as you move through the poses. Once you have a basic knowledge of the location and the functionality of each chakra and are able to connect yoga asanas and the chakra system together, you can heal your body and mind more efficiently. Through a consistent chakra yoga practice over time,

you can improve your quality of life by feeling lighter and less anxious, with more flexibility and strength. It is a way of life that takes commitment, but it is definitely worth the time and effort.

In this book, you will learn the basics about the chakras, such as their individual locations in the body, what they govern in terms of your physical well-being, and what it feels like when there is an issue that needs to be addressed, such as a blockage or lack of energy in that area. You will also learn how to heal problems that may come up and achieve balance throughout your body. There are guided yoga poses and sequences that you can practice on your own, which is a great place to begin your journey in the exploration of chakra yoga.

While chakra yoga is a great way to heal your body and mind from many ailments, it is best to practice it in conjunction with consulting medical professionals. Chakra yoga is an excellent supplementary tool for improving your overall health and well-being, and it can be used along with treatments your physician prescribes or recommends. As long as you consult your doctor, listen to your body, and be kind to yourself, you will achieve a great amount of healing and balance.

PART 1

CONNECTING *the* MIND *and* BODY

CHAPTER 1

the harmony of chakra and yoga

In this chapter, we will learn about the chakras, what they are, and how they affect the mind and body overall. We will discuss the way energy flows through the chakras that are dispersed throughout the body, and what happens when there is too much or too little energy in one area. We will learn about the strong connection between the chakras and yoga, and how a well-balanced yoga practice can aid in discovering—and balancing—the chakras.

Vibrant Health and Spiritual Awakening

The word "chakra" directly translates to "wheel," and the system of chakras refers to the centers of energy distributed throughout the body. This is the body's energy system, where we get our power and vitality. Each chakra has its own unique location, and there are 7 primary chakras along with 21 minor chakras.

Each chakra has multiple layers of energy, which work together to contribute to the chakras' overall health. The chakras are interconnected and work together as a collective unit. If one chakra is out of balance, it is likely that the others around it are compensating for that imbalance. It is very important to pay attention to the chakras and acknowledge their presence in your body to avoid imbalances and blockages in multiple areas.

As you will learn more in depth, these imbalances or blockages can manifest as a variety of unwanted physical and emotional ailments. Balancing the chakras helps with the overall flow of energy throughout the body, which makes us feel lighter, happier, and healthier.

The Flow of Divine Energy

Energy typically flows consistently throughout the chakras all day, every day. It is powering your body and your life. It is what is responsible for getting you out of bed in the morning and moving you along throughout your day. It is our life force, and it keeps us going. We need it to survive.

If you wake up full of energy and ready to start your day, it is likely that you have free-flowing, balanced energy throughout your chakras. This balance will carry you through the day and allow you to achieve your goals, enjoy your life, have fulfilling relationships with others, and fully accept and love yourself.

Far too often, we find ourselves suffering from physical or mental pain. While pain is a part of life and does happen every so often, it does not have to run our lives. If our energy is openly flowing, we will feel a noticeable difference in our overall health and well-being.

This energy or life force is called *prana*, and when it flows freely through the chakra system, we feel healthy, light, and balanced. It is a really great feeling that unfortunately many of us do not get to experience on a regular basis. This is why becoming aware of the chakras within our bodies is so important.

The Healing Power of Yoga

A well-balanced yoga practice can be a remarkably helpful tool in achieving health and wellness in the body, mind, and spirit. "Yoga" directly translates to "yoke," and it can also mean "unify" or "unite." This unification signifies connectivity of mind, body, and spirit, which can be further recognized over time through a consistent yoga practice. A well-balanced yoga practice consists of breathing techniques, meditation, and asana practice—the physical postures of yoga, which is what usually comes to mind when most people think of yoga.

We practice yoga to revitalize and rejuvenate our body and mind, which assists in connecting with the spirit. Although people often turn to yoga for such reasons as weight loss, injury recovery, or relaxation, yoga is much more than that and can be a vital tool for achieving overall health.

Yoga can also greatly aid in unblocking, activating, and healing the chakras. Practicing yoga gives us insight we would not be able to achieve in other ways. This internal awareness is crucial for recognizing each chakra individually and as a connected unit, which helps us understand what is happening within our own bodies.

Yoga can be practiced by everyone, regardless of age, gender, weight, or any other factor one might feel is holding them back. While yoga can be more challenging for some, it does not look the same on everyone. It is very important to not compare yourself to others when practicing yoga because your body is likely to look very different from your neighbor's body. It is important to understand that modifications can and should be made to accommodate *your* body, and there is nothing wrong with modifying a yoga pose to fit your specific needs.

It is also important to note that a well-balanced yoga practice involves both passive and active forms of yoga—this is often referred to as yin and yang. It is just as important to practice the more passive and restorative postures in yoga as it is to practice the more active and invigorating ones. In this book, I will speak a great deal about achieving balance, and this aspect of yoga is no different. In order to counterbalance the rigor of an active yoga posture or routine, one must incorporate a passive, restorative aspect to the practice as well.

The key to achieving the most out of your yoga practice is to practice consistently. You will not see changes and results overnight. You can achieve many great things through yoga, including a healthier and happier life, but you will not see results if you do not put in regular work.

Practicing the Essential Poses

In this book, you will find detailed explanations of yoga poses and sequences to help you connect with and awaken your chakra-healing power. I explain each pose, and modification options if applicable, in a simple manner. The yoga sequences are easy to follow and specifically designed to aid in your journey toward a healthy and balanced mind and body.

In addition to the yoga asana instructions, you will find supplementary tips and activities to incorporate into your yoga practice, such as breathing techniques and meditation exercises. The combination of physical and mental yoga techniques is vital to a healthy and well-rounded practice. Each yoga posture, tip, and activity corresponds to a specific chakra.

It is important to understand which poses are closely connected to each chakra so you can customize your yoga practice to fit your needs. In this book, you will be guided through all aspects of a chakra yoga practice. It will allow you to integrate your own personalized chakra yoga routine into your daily life.

PRACTICE COMPASSION

YOGA CAN HELP in achieving inner peace and overall healing of the mind and body. However, this wonderful gift does not come easily. Consistency in a yoga practice is the key element to achieving your health and wellness goals. As a yoga teacher, I see it time and time again: A beginner yoga student tries one class and feels great afterward but does not commit to practicing regularly. Then they do not understand why they aren't seeing any results. A commitment to consistency and focus will provide you with the results you are looking to achieve and then some.

While putting in the work is crucial to reaching goals, it is also very important to practice self-compassion. Being kind to yourself is just as important as practicing regularly. This means if you are ill or unable to practice, it is totally fine to resume your regular practice when you are feeling better. You can always modify poses to suit your specific needs at any time throughout your practice, all the way from the beginner to advanced levels. Never feel ashamed or put yourself down for needing to modify a pose—everyone's body is different.

Having a combination of determination, focus, compassion, and patience will help you achieve your health and wellness goals over time through a consistent and well-rounded chakra yoga practice.

Searching for Well-Being

A harmonious chakra feels refreshed and revitalized, and you can feel the energy flowing effortlessly through it within your body. This effortless flow of *prana* is what we are all looking to achieve, yet this can be hard to come by. Energy flow allows you to feel free both inside and outside your body. A free-flowing chakra gives you plenty of energy and power in the area it is connected to. It also provides that area with a balanced sense of peace and calm.

A blocked chakra often feels just like that: blocked. It feels as if the energy is stuck and stagnant, and it can prevent a full range of motion in that particular area of the body. A blocked chakra stops a balanced flow of *prana* to the surrounding chakras, causing problems in those areas as well. It can make your body feel stiff in that spot, or it can bring forth physical health issues, such as headaches, stomach pain, and joint pain, depending on the chakra. It can also generate emotional or mental health issues, such as anxiety, depression, or phobias, depending on the affected chakra. These can be just as debilitating as physical ailments, if not more so.

As discussed previously, following a dedicated chakra yoga practice takes time in order to achieve results. You must tune in to your body, commit to a consistent practice, and focus on the specific chakras and areas that are blocked and need attention.

Similar to going to the doctor for an annual checkup and tending to our general health, it is important to care for the alignment of our chakras. Even though you may feel fine and have no obvious ailments that need immediate attention, taking care of the chakras and making sure they stay balanced and aligned is key to living a healthy and balanced life.

Balance and Healing

An overactive chakra means there is too much energy flowing into that area. This can be caused by a blockage in a surrounding chakra, or sometimes a trauma to that area pulls in more energy to expedite the healing process. Although the idea of having more energy seems like a good thing, it can do more harm than good. As you will see in the following chapter, a surplus of energy in a certain chakra can cause problems as well.

An underactive chakra does not have enough energy flowing to it, which can also be caused by a blockage in a surrounding chakra that doesn't allow a sufficient amount of the body's supply of energy to reach it. This tends to make the chakra take on a more passive role in the body, and as a result it is not able to work in conjunction with the other chakras.

This causes sluggishness and lack of movement in the affected area.

As I mentioned earlier, a balanced chakra feels free, revitalized, energized, and at peace. It has just enough energy to support that area of the body in functioning properly and working with its connected parts. Achieving a balanced chakra system as a whole is our goal.

Since the body and mind are so closely connected and intertwined, it is important to note that finding balance in one often results in relief in the other as well. If an emotional or mental health issue is resolved and balance is restored, we often find that our corresponding physical issues alleviate or disappear completely.

This can be surprising to many, as it is a common misconception that the body and mind should be treated as separate entities. This could not be further from the truth, and discovering more about your chakras is a perfect way to see how.

A chakra yoga practice that is customized to suit your personal needs can enable you to achieve balance in the chakras and overall healing. This can provide short-term pain relief and heal severely neglected emotional issues, which can help you live a better life and feel good now. A balanced chakra system through a chakra yoga practice can also provide long-term benefits that can be seen in your health as you age.

CHAPTER 2

discovering the chakras

In this chapter, we will look at each chakra and learn how to differentiate between them. We will explore how to understand the chakras and work with them in order to achieve healing within the body. We will also learn how to become more in tune with the body and how to figure out if the chakras are blocked. Discovering more about the chakras is a great beginning to a chakra yoga practice.

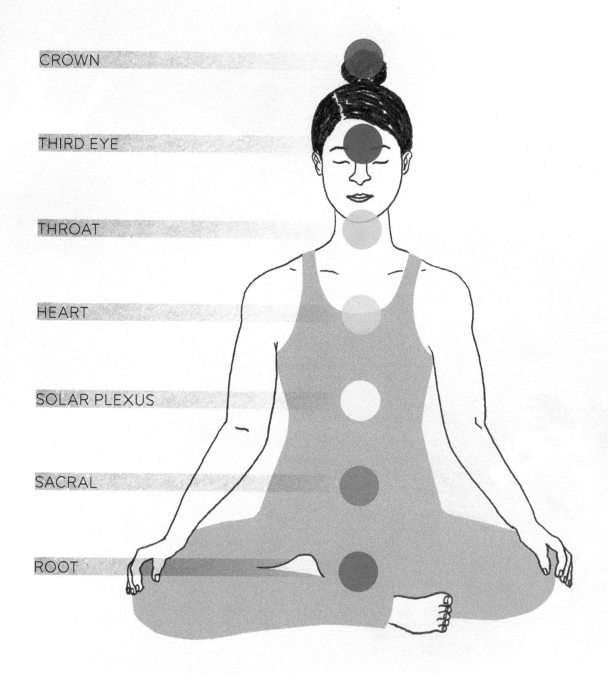

CROWN

THIRD EYE

THROAT

HEART

SOLAR PLEXUS

SACRAL

ROOT

Becoming One with the Chakra System

As we learned earlier, the chakras are a system of energy wheels that power your body as a whole. They are deeply connected and intertwined with one another, and when one is off-balance, it can knock the others off as well. There is a constant supply of *prana* that flows through the chakras individually and as a system. Each chakra has a location in the body, a Sanskrit name, an element, an affirmation for healing, positive and negative archetypes, and physical and emotional dysfunctions. Balancing the entire chakra system is not an easy task, but working toward creating balance is definitely worthwhile, as it can provide you with a healthier and happier life.

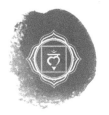

ROOT CHAKRA

Location: The base of the spine (coccyx), the pelvic floor muscles (perineum)

Names: Muladhara

Element: Earth

Affirmation: I am grounded, safe, and secure. My needs are always met, and I live a life of abundance.

Mantra: LAM

Archetypes (positive and negative):

- A positive root chakra archetype feels strong, secure, energetic, and healthy, and is fully able to give and receive love.
- A negative root chakra archetype often feels insecure and a lack of control in all aspects of life. They are not self-sufficient and have trouble receiving love from others.

Physical dysfunctions: Dysfunction in the colon, bladder, or bowels; leg, knee, or foot problems; issues with the prostate

Emotional issues: Anxiety disorders, phobias

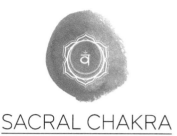

SACRAL CHAKRA

Location: The lower abdomen from the genitals up to just below the navel
Names: Svadhisthana
Element: Water
Affirmation: I am emotionally balanced, and I have comfortable and safe relationships with those who love me.
Mantra: VAM
Archetypes (positive and negative):
- A positive sacral chakra archetype is generally an optimist who looks at all aspects of life with a positive attitude. They can appreciate the good things in life and have a healthy relationship with eating and food.
- A negative sacral chakra archetype lives in a relentless world of self-pity and does not feel appreciated for the things they do for others. They may also have a negative relationship with food consumption.

Physical dysfunctions: Issues with the reproductive system, urinary tract and kidney infections, constipation, lower-back pain
Emotional issues: Eating disorders, depression

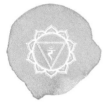

SOLAR PLEXUS CHAKRA

Location: The solar plexus (a.k.a. celiac plexus) at the center of the abdomen, above the navel and below the chest
Names: Manipura
Element: Fire
Affirmation: I am a powerful, confident, and graceful person, and I am fully in control of my life.
Mantra: RAM
Archetypes (positive and negative):
- A positive solar plexus archetype has strong willpower and the ability to see things through and achieve their goals.
- A negative solar plexus archetype needs constant validation from others and has no sense of individuality. They often turn to self-sabotage in the pursuit of achieving goals.

Physical dysfunctions: Digestive disorders, gall bladder and liver issues, ulcers, diabetes
Emotional issues: Addiction, codependency

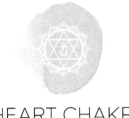

HEART CHAKRA

Location: Near the heart and lungs in the cardiac plexus, or the chest area

Names: Anahata

Element: Air

Affirmation: I am worthy and able to give and receive love unconditionally, and I feel a sense of peace and calm within my heart.

Mantra: YAM

Archetypes (positive and negative):

• A positive heart chakra archetype is very trusting, empathetic, and forgiving, and loves others and oneself unconditionally.

• A negative heart chakra archetype does not allow oneself to fully give and receive love due to fear of rejection and getting hurt. They push people away and are jealous, untrusting, and judgmental.

Physical dysfunctions: Dysfunctional immune system, heart problems, breast cancer, respiratory and lung issues, upper-back pain

Emotional issues: Post-traumatic stress disorder, depression, grief

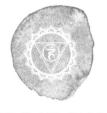

THROAT CHAKRA

Location: The throat, neck, and shoulder area

Names: Vishuddha

Element: Ether

Affirmation: I am able to communicate my truth clearly and with ease. I am a good listener, while also allowing others to hear my voice and honor my feelings.

Mantra: HAM

Archetypes (positive and negative):

• A positive throat chakra archetype is clearly able to express their feelings and thoughts. They are not afraid to speak up and be heard.

• A negative throat chakra archetype holds in their feelings and cannot express needs, thoughts, or fears.

Physical dysfunctions: Thyroid problems, sore throat, neck pain, dental issues

Emotional issues: Social anxiety, glossophobia (fear of speech), extreme diffidence

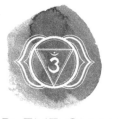

THIRD-EYE CHAKRA

Location: The center of the forehead between the eyebrows

Names: Ajna

Element: Light

Affirmation: My thoughts are clear, and my mind is healthy. I trust myself and my intuition to guide me in the right direction.

Mantra: AUM (a.k.a. OM)

Archetypes (positive and negative):

• A positive third-eye chakra archetype is creative, intuitive, and trusts their intuition to guide them in the right direction.

• A negative third-eye chakra archetype is a know-it-all who always has to be right. They are very opinionated and at times suppress their true feelings.

Physical dysfunctions: Sinus issues, vision problems, headaches, insomnia

Emotional issues: Excessive feelings of being overwhelmed and anxious, lack of mental clarity

CROWN CHAKRA

Location: Slightly above the top of the head

Names: Sahasrara

Element: Thought

Affirmation: I am complete and perfect as I am. I feel connected to a higher source, and I am confident in my life's purpose.

Mantra: AUM (specifically the silence after AUM)

Archetypes (positive and negative):

• A positive crown chakra archetype is fully connected to a higher power and is grateful, humble, and loves all beings.

• A negative crown chakra archetype is self-obsessed, arrogant, and proud, and often boasts about their achievements without modesty.

Physical dysfunctions: Frequent migraines, headaches, fatigue

Emotional issues: Obsessive issues, addiction, delusion

THE MINOR CHAKRAS

The seven chakras just described are the primary ones, which are all a part of the major chakra system and our body's main source of energy and power. There are also 21 supplementary chakras that are dispersed throughout the body as smaller acupoints complementing each of the major chakras. This is the minor chakra system.

While we will focus mainly on the seven major chakras over the course of this book, it is important to acknowledge the existence of the minor chakras, as they surround each major chakra. You can think of the minor chakras as fine-tuning, while the major chakras are the foundation and basis of the body's energy. Becoming aware of the seven major power centers in your body is the first step toward growth and healing, and the simple acknowledgment that there is more to the story will be a great tool as you move further along in your practice.

FEELING YOUR PRANA

A SIMPLE EXERCISE to connect with your chakras as a whole is to do a *yoga nidra* body scan while lying in Savasana (a.k.a. Corpse Pose).

Lie flat on your back on the floor or on a yoga mat. Move your legs slightly apart and place your hands on the floor by your sides with your palms facing up. Relax your limbs completely. Bring your gaze upward so your spine is straight, and close your eyes. Breathe through your nose and begin to deepen your breathing. Focus on your inhales and exhales for the first minute or so to draw your attention inward.

Once you feel a sense of quiet within your body and mind, begin scanning your body. Start with your feet and gradually work your way up to the ankles, lower legs, upper legs, pelvis, hips, lower back, upper back, hands, arms, shoulders, neck, and finally your head. Spend a good amount of time—whatever feels appropriate for you—on each body part and keep breathing. Notice and acknowledge how each body part is feeling, and without moving that body part, just observe how it feels to you and then move on to the next.

Once you have scanned the entire body, feel the *prana* flowing through each and every part that you just observed. You may feel a slight tingling sensation throughout the body, which is normal. Practicing this meditation allows you to find where there may be chakra imbalances or blockages, helping inform your chakra yoga practice.

Blocked Chakras

A blocked chakra is when energy, or *prana*, is not able to flow through that specific center of energy. To give you a better idea of what it might look like, let's compare the system of chakras in your body to a series of connected highways, and *prana* to the cars on those highways.

If all the highway lanes are open and clear, then traffic can flow smoothly and efficiently. But what if some of the lanes are closed off? This would prevent cars from flowing smoothly along the highway as a whole, which would ultimately cause a traffic jam. The cars stuck in this traffic jam will get to their destination eventually, because there are still some open lanes on the highway, but they will get there a lot more slowly. And even though there are lanes closed on one highway, that also affects traffic on other highways, as they are all connected. The same goes for the chakras in your body. If one chakra is blocked, *prana* is still able to flow through, just not as freely. This also affects other chakras, because they have to compensate for the lack of energy, or buildup of energy, due to the blockage.

A blocked chakra can cause physical and emotional issues in the corresponding area of the body. For instance, if you have a blocked throat chakra in the neck, the lack of free-flowing energy through that chakra could cause physical issues, such as neck pain or a sore throat. Since your body, mind, and spirit are all connected as well, physical issues can also manifest as mental and emotional problems, or vice versa.

Chakras can become blocked for a variety of reasons, including physical and emotional trauma, mental and physical abuse, addiction, surgery, and not taking care of your basic needs (sleep, nutrition, exercise, hygiene, and so on). These issues can often be subtle and tend to appear without us even recognizing that there is a problem.

Detecting Blocked Chakras

Your body communicates a blocked chakra through a physical or emotional ailment that comes to the surface. These problems are your body's way of telling you that something is off. Physical and emotional symptoms will be different with each person, so comparing yourself to someone else is not the best option for discovering your own personal blocked chakras.

It is necessary to recognize the areas where you are blocked and that you need to address. Here are some ways you can get more in tune with your body in order to identify blocked chakras:

1. **Sit quietly and breathe.** This activity can also be seen as a form of meditation, except you do not necessarily have to focus solely on the breath. Try sitting down, either on the floor in a cross-legged position or in a chair with your feet flat on the floor, and just be with yourself.

2. **Body-scanning exercise.** There is a yogic technique called *yoga nidra* (see "Feeling Your Prana" sidebar, page 16). In this exercise, you lie flat on your back with your eyes closed and mentally scan along your body, starting with your feet and working your way up. You can use a guided *yoga nidra* meditation or do it on your own, spending three to five deep breaths on each body part, or however long you feel is needed.

3. **Walking meditation.** Sometimes it is helpful to listen to your body while moving. Try taking a long, scenic, slow walk through the woods or a quiet park. You can put your headphones on and listen to some gentle ambient music without words, but it is best if you are able to do this in silence. As you are walking, you can direct your attention inward and scan your body in order to listen to what it is telling you.

4. **Journaling exercises.** Try sitting down in a quiet place and freely writing whatever comes to mind in response to the following questions: Is there a problem? What is the problem? Where is the problem? What does it feel like? What caused it? You can spend however long you would like discussing each question and working through it with yourself.

5. **Massage or self-massage.** Having a massage performed on you or massaging out your own muscles using a foam roller or yoga therapy balls can be quite helpful in discovering areas where you are tight and holding tension.

Be patient with yourself when trying to discover your blockages. Some blocked chakras are subtle and not easy to detect, but it is possible to use these techniques to listen to what your body is trying to tell you. If you listen closely enough, you will be able to uncover any blocked chakras and address the problem at the source.

Unblocking Chakras

The focal point of this book is practicing the yoga asanas and how they can help you discover, balance, and harmonize your body's chakras. However, there are several ways to unblock the chakras, and you can use one or more of these techniques to complement the others.

Meditation is a major part of a well-balanced yoga practice, and it is also a great way to focus your attention on a specific chakra.

Another method is having a Reiki session performed on you by a professional. Using Reiki to move your body's energy around is an excellent way to aid the flow of *prana* through the body. This is great if it is incorporated into your yoga practice and done before or after you practice.

Some believe in the power of crystals, and there are certain crystals specifically assigned to each chakra, which you can place on or near that area of the body during meditation.

You can also use aromatherapy to unblock your chakras, as there are specific scents assigned to each chakra.

CHAPTER 3

beginning your chakra yoga practice

In this chapter, we will learn the best methods for deciding which chakra or chakras to focus on healing. We will go over how to get in touch with the body and understand which parts of it need more attention. From there, we can figure out where to direct that attention and successfully guide a yoga practice toward those areas.

Navigating Chakra Yoga

Approach the chakra yoga practice by first discovering where your blockages are, and then learning which poses and sequences balance the chakra that you need to work on. This will help inform your practice and give you a guided and structured approach that will be more effective in healing you faster. Once you have decided what you would like to focus on, put a plan into place that will help you work toward achieving your goals.

Also, be aware that as you become more in touch with your body, you may notice imbalances in multiple chakras. You might want to work on everything at once, but be cautious. As with most things, it is best to focus on one thing at a time. You may move through a yoga sequence that addresses different chakras, giving you a full-body experience; however, if you have a specific goal of unlocking your root chakra, for instance, then start with that and focus most of your energy there first.

It is also good practice to start from the bottom and work your way up. As discussed in the previous chapter, there are seven major chakras. The root chakra is known as the first major chakra because it is at the bottom of the spine and acts as the foundation for the rest of the chakras. If you are looking to balance more than one of your chakras, it is best to begin at the lowest one. This will create a ripple effect as healing works its way up the system along the spine, building a solid foundation for all the chakras to heal and thrive.

Practice as often as you are able to, but at least once a week. If you can practice daily, go for it. Start with one session and try to fit more into your schedule as time goes on. You will likely find yourself wanting to increase the frequency of your sessions because of how good you feel afterward.

Creating Your Own Practice

Since you are reading this book, it is likely that you are looking to form an at-home yoga practice and ritual for yourself. Creating a dedicated yoga space in your home is a great way to generate habit and a sense of desire to get onto your mat and practice regularly. This space should be aesthetically pleasing to you and calming for your mind. It should help the flow of creativity and inspire you not only in your yoga practice, but in other areas of your life as well. If you do not have a designated space in your home where you can keep your yoga props out at all times, store them, and when you take them out for practice, you are creating a ritual—a tradition—that you will ultimately find a regular sense of comfort in.

I will go into the necessary yoga props in a bit more detail later on, but first I'll mention that it is really nice to have a dedicated yoga mat that is only yours. This yoga mat is your sacred place, where you can come to heal your mind, body, and spirit. It should be treated well, cleaned, and stored in a protective way. It is also common for people to use the public mats at their studio or gym where they attend classes. While this is a fine option if you are short on space at home, it is not ideal if you are looking to build a personal chakra yoga practice for yourself and your overall healing. I highly encourage you to invest in and take good care of your own yoga mat for your practice.

As you begin to develop your own practice, you will come to find that your yoga mat is your special zone, an area that brings you joy. I have had the same yoga mat for about five years, and it is still going strong. The dusty pink color brings me joy every time I look at it, and the material feels good when it comes into contact with my skin. I have great affinity for my mat, and I almost think of it as an old friend who is always there for me no matter what is going on

in my life. I believe that everyone should have the same kind of relationship with their yoga mat because it strengthens the special bond you have with your yoga practice.

Speaking of bonding with your practice: It is important to not only set up a designated yoga space, but also to establish a routine for yourself. Consider what you would like to accomplish and use that as motivation to keep coming back to your practice. Goal setting—to have a clear picture in your mind about what you would like to achieve—is so important in all aspects of life, and your yoga practice is no different. Goals will help you establish your practice on your own terms and stay motivated to keep coming back to your mat.

LISTENING TO YOUR BODY

This book will guide you step-by-step through the yoga poses and sequences to take the guesswork out of what you should be doing when practicing the yoga asanas. This will aid your practice, but it is no substitute for an in-person yoga teacher and your knowledge about your own body. If you find yourself struggling, or if something does not feel good, then move out of that pose; do not force yourself. Use modifications and yoga props where needed to help the pose feel better in *your* body. Always use your body as a guide, and listen to its cues. While it is great to challenge yourself to grow and improve, forcing yourself into a yoga pose that you are not ready for is never the answer. There are ways to work your way up to achieving the full expression of the poses, and you must be patient with yourself.

It is important to recognize the difference between the good type of pain, which is helping you get stronger, and the bad type of pain, which is causing your body harm. If you experience sharp pain in a joint (where two bones are fitted together), then move out of the pose immediately. Dull pain in the middle of the muscles is okay as your muscles stretch and gain flexibility. It is important to get in tune with your body by following the guidelines outlined in the previous chapter to help you understand what your body is trying to tell you. Your body is very smart, and you can trust its signals. You just have to know how to interpret the messages.

Holding Poses

In this book, I will advise a suggested amount of time to hold each pose within a sequence, but it is also important to listen to your body and make that decision for yourself. As you deepen your practice and get more accustomed to practicing yoga regularly, you will begin to develop an intuition about how long to stay in each pose.

For a hatha or vinyasa yoga class, you should hold the poses for three to five deep and full breaths, in and out through the nose. For a yin or restorative practice, you will hold the poses for much longer, generally three to five minutes each, which translates to 20 to 30 deep and full breaths. But these are not hard-and-fast rules. At times, your teacher or the yoga sequence you are following may advise you to hold a certain pose for a bit longer to emphasize a certain movement, or they may just pass through a pose more quickly. It depends on many different factors, including the class style, the purpose or theme of that class or sequence, and the teacher.

You can also look for signals from your body to let you know when it is time to exit a pose. As I mentioned earlier, you will need to listen to your body and understand which types of pain are good and which are bad. Your body will always want to choose the path of least resistance, so understanding that some types of pain are good is crucial to your growth. When in doubt, if the pain is too intense, come out of it until you have a better grasp on what you should and should not be feeling. This wisdom will come over time, so as always, be patient with yourself and continue to practice regularly and consistently.

LEAVING YOUR COMFORT ZONE

Many people in the yoga world speak about finding your "edge" in the pose and taking your body there before coming out of it. You will learn more about where your personal edge is over time as you progress through your yoga practice. A good guideline for finding where that edge is for yourself is understanding when your body's survival mode tends to kick in. This is the moment when your body generally gets tired and wants to choose the path of least resistance. Once you realize that the pain or discomfort you may be experiencing is not the bad type of pain and you are able to stay in the pose without causing harm to your body, then you can acknowledge and move past your edge.

When you reach and move past your edge, not only does your body improve, get stronger, and gain flexibility, but you also experience the change of energy flow within your chakras. Change must occur in order to achieve balance in your chakras, especially if you have a blockage in a certain area. You will learn this over time through your personal journey, so trust the process and be patient with yourself.

Harnessing Your Breath

The breath is a vital aspect of a yoga practice and moving through the yoga poses, and it can also be used as a tool to support and advance your practice. There are specific breathing techniques and exercises that you can do to feel relaxed, gain energy, feel grounded, and more. However, you can simply incorporate breathing into your asana practice as well to help you feel better in the poses and improve within your body.

The life force of your body is your breath, and therefore "*prana*," "breath," and "energy" can be used interchangeably. While there is a difference between energy and breath in terms of physicality and location within the body, breath is simply the release or intake of energy. When you inhale, you are bringing energy and power in, and that energy continues to flow through the body and the chakras. When you exhale, you are releasing energy out of the body, continuing the pathway of the flow of energy.

Breath can be used as a tool to help you feel more relaxed and slow down your heart rate if you are feeling anxious. It can also be used to deepen a stretch. As you exhale, you can gently ease your body a bit deeper into the stretch, coming to your edge and continuing to breathe through any discomfort. You can also use your breath to connect to your subconscious during meditation. The act of focusing on your breath brings your attention to what is happening inside your body and allows you to observe how you are feeling on the inside. As you get to know yourself and your body on a deeper level, you will also build a deeper relationship with your breath and gain a greater understanding of it.

GRANTHIS (KNOTS)

Granthi translates to "knot," and it refers to the concept that blocked energy is restrictive and difficult to untie. If you find that you have blocked chakras, you will likely be dealing with *granthis*. These restrict the passage of *prana* throughout the body and can be caused by a variety of happenings in your life. They result in you becoming stuck in your ways, not allowing yourself to be open to new possibilities. These can be general or more specific, depending on the area where the *granthi* exists and what caused it. There are ways to release your *granthis* that are detailed later, and you can incorporate them into your chakra yoga practice.

BANDHAS (LOCKS)

Practicing the *bandhas* ("locks") can help in releasing your *granthis* and aid in your quest to unblock your chakras.

Bandhas help you shift and move your *prana* to different areas of the body where your *granthis* and chakra blocks may be restricting its access. There are four *bandhas* in the body that you can incorporate into your chakra yoga practice:

1. **Mula Bandha.** This is the root lock, and to execute it, you must activate and squeeze in the muscles in the perineum area at the first chakra, Muladhara. This is commonly known as a Kegel, and it is often practiced to strengthen vaginal muscles before and after childbirth.

2. **Uddiyana Bandha.** This lock happens in your abdominal area, and it is the act of drawing all the organs in your abdomen upward as you bend forward. You can rest your hands on your legs as you are bringing those muscles and organs up and in.

3. **Jalandhara Bandha.** This lock takes place in the neck area, and it can be done by sitting up tall in a cross-legged position with your hands on your legs. Draw your sternum up and your chin down to a place where they meet each other halfway.

4. **Maha Bandha.** This is the act of completing all three of the previously mentioned locks simultaneously as you sit in a cross-legged position and firmly anchor your hands down onto your legs.

Practicing these *bandhas* and holding them for as long as you are able to will make you stronger and aid in the flow of energy throughout the body.

RELEASING YOUR PAST

At times, as we begin to open and balance our chakras, many past traumas and tensions can get brought to the forefront. As humans, we often suppress traumatic and painful experiences that have happened in our past to avoid feeling the pain. As I mentioned before, our minds and bodies usually choose the path of least resistance, and sometimes avoiding emotional pain is a part of that path.

While it may be more comfortable to avoid pain, it is important to lean into it and push through so we can get past it and move on. If this happens to you during your chakra yoga practice, sit with whatever feelings come up for you and observe them. If you need to cry, it is absolutely okay. Do not be afraid to let it out and release whatever you are feeling. You can even incorporate journaling about the experience, which often helps get the thoughts and feelings out.

Once you observe your thoughts and feelings, acknowledge that whatever you're pulling up is not happening now; it is just a memory. Also acknowledge that your thoughts are not you, they do not define you, and you can observe them without judgment before you watch them fade away. It may take a bit of time to feel better, but you must not repress those feelings again once they resurface. Be sure to take the time to release them properly and work through them by way of observation, journaling, and emotional release before moving forward.

AWAKENING THE CHAKRAS THROUGH DANCE

YOU CAN USE the act of dance to unblock and balance your chakras as well. Simply moving the area of a specific chakra in a rhythmic way can activate the flow of energy. While you can certainly dance freely to your own beat, there are also aspects of dance that you can incorporate into your dancing to help with the flow of *prana* throughout the body.

Nritta: This is the dramatic aspect of dance. It adds a story or feeling to your movement, which can be seen through the expressions on your face.

Nritya: This is a form of miming or interpretive dance. Let's say you are dancing to a song with lyrics. Nritya would be the act of acting out the words with your movements, like a form of charades but with flow and rhythm.

Natya: This is the physical act of dance itself. It is the rhythmic movement performed by the body without interpretation.

Combining all three of these aspects, or categories, of dance can be a great way to aid in the flow of *prana* throughout the chakras, move through any chakra blocks, and have a bit of fun.

Preparing for Your Practice

It is now time to prepare for your chakra yoga practice. With your newfound understanding of the foundations of what a chakra yoga practice means and what it can do for you, you should be able to create the right mind-set, surroundings, and tools for yourself to begin your journey. As you begin to get more in touch with your body, pinpoint what areas you would like to focus on. This will help you craft your chakra yoga practice using the tips in this chapter and upcoming chapters as well.

WEAR COMFORTABLE CLOTHING

Be sure you feel comfortable in the clothes you wear during your yoga practice. Avoid tight elastic bands and clothing, which will prevent you from being able to move to your fullest potential. Also, avoid clothes that are too loose fitting, as extra fabric can impede your movements or get caught.

GET THE RIGHT PROPS

As mentioned before, it is greatly beneficial to get a personal yoga mat that is only for you to help establish a special ritual and a sacred place for your practice. You can also use yoga blocks, yoga straps, yoga blankets, and yoga bolsters to help facilitate the poses. If a pose or a pose modification requires a yoga prop, it will be specified along with a substitute option.

SET UP YOUR SPACE

Creating a safe and special place for your yoga practice that is aesthetically pleasing can be a great motivator to keep you coming back to your mat on a regular basis.

SET YOUR MIND FOR SUCCESS

And finally, setting your mind for success is key. Have your goals in mind before you begin and use your clear plan of action to build your personalized practice. Be kind to yourself and practice self-compassion as you move through your journey, and understand that it takes a great amount of time and effort to achieve your goals and see results. So, get on your yoga mat and keep up the great work!

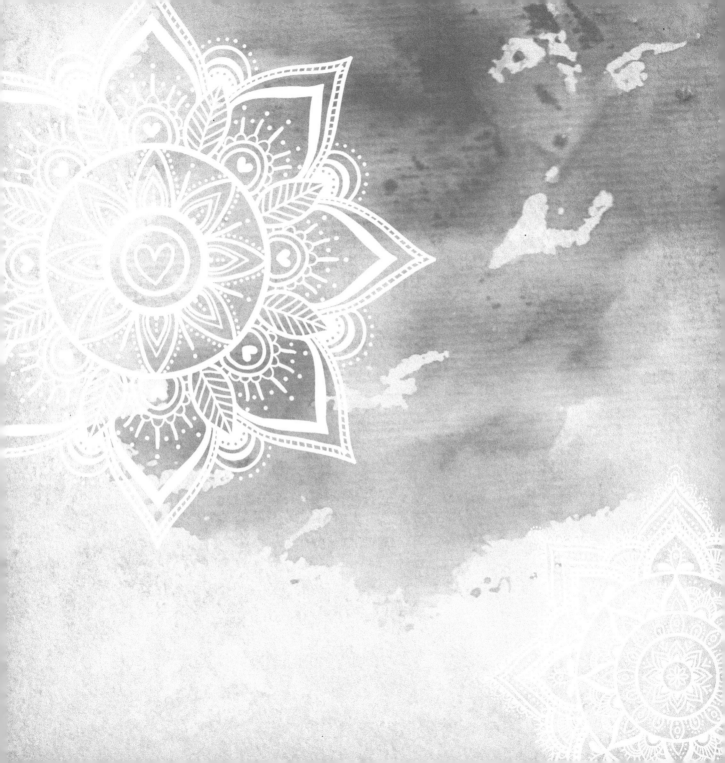

PART 2

HEALING THROUGH CHAKRA YOGA

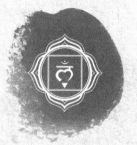

root chakra

This chakra is located at the base of the spine and the pelvic floor area, and it governs our basic needs. With a balanced root chakra, we should feel secure and stable in our lives, from our physical needs (food and water) to our emotional needs (stability and balance). Yoga can help balance this chakra by building a connection between us and that area, as well as releasing tension and building strength in the surrounding muscles.

Siddhasana Accomplished Pose

This simple pose is often done during meditation and at the beginning or end of a yoga class. With your heels pointed toward the root chakra, it will help you draw energy and attention toward that area.

Props: Mat, blanket

Precautions: Use caution or avoid this pose if you have recently had a knee or hip-joint injury or suffer from chronic pain in either of these areas.

Benefits:
- Promotes hip flexibility
- Helps you feel grounded
- Comfortable seat for meditation

Instructions:

1. Come to a seat on the floor and sit up tall on the two sit bones at the bottom of your pelvis.

2. Bend both of your legs and bring your heels in toward the pelvis, bringing one foot in front of the other and aligning both heels with your pubic bone.

3. Bring your hands to a resting position with your palms facing up on your legs.

4. Inhale and lengthen your spine; exhale, spread your shoulders apart, and soften your ribs in toward one another.

5. Hold for as long as you are able to or as instructed, if you are practicing this pose as part of a sequence.

TIP: Place a folded yoga blanket under your hips and sit on the rounded edge of the blanket to promote a forward tilt of your pelvis. This alleviates any gripping you may feel in your hip sockets and knee joints.

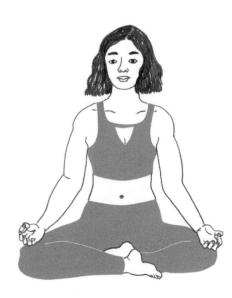

Anjaneyasana Low Lunge (Variation with the Knee Down)

This straightforward pose opens the root chakra and the surrounding muscles and joints.

Prop: Mat

Precautions: Use caution or avoid this pose if you have recently had a knee or hip injury or suffer from chronic pain in either of these areas.

Benefits:
- Promotes hip flexibility
- Stretches the quadriceps
- Relieves tension and stress

Instructions:

1. Begin on your hands and knees and bring one bent leg toward the front of your mat, placing the bottom of your foot on the floor between your hands.

2. The knee of the front leg should be directly above the foot and tracking in line with the second and third toes.

3. Bring the shin of the back leg and the top of the back foot down on the ground behind you.

4. The hands should be on the ground, framing the front foot, and your gaze should be on the ground between your hands, keeping the spine long.

5. Inhale and lengthen the spine; exhale and gently press the hips down toward the ground.

6. Hold for three to five breaths.

7. To come out of this pose, press into the ground with your hands and bring the front leg back under your hips in a hands-and-knees position.

8. Repeat on the other side.

TIP: If you are feeling pressure or pain on the knee joint of the back leg, you can fold your yoga mat over to create a double layer of cushion under that joint.

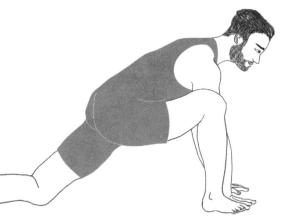

Baddha Konasana Bound-Angle Pose

This seated forward fold will stretch the hips in an externally rotated position, which is another great way to open up that area. It is also very calming and will help center your energy toward the root chakra.

Props: Mat, blanket, blocks

Precautions: Use caution or avoid this pose if you have recently had a lower-back, knee, or hip injury or suffer from chronic pain in any of these areas.

Benefits:
- Promotes external rotation of the hips
- Calms the body and mind
- Releases tension and stress

Instructions:

1. Begin in a seated position on the floor, sitting tall on the two sit bones at the bottom of your pelvis.

2. Bend both legs and bring the bottoms of your feet toward your body to meet sole-to-sole at the center line.

3. Hold your ankles with your hands; your knees should be out to either side of you.

4. Inhale and lengthen the spine, then exhale and fold the torso forward.

5. For a deeper hip opening, while you are bending forward, bring your elbows to both knees and gently press the knees down toward the floor.

6. Hold for three to five breaths.

7. To come out of this pose, on an inhale, slowly bring the torso back upright and release the legs from their position.

TIP: Place a folded yoga blanket under your hips and sit on the rounded edge of the blanket to promote a forward tilt of your pelvis. This alleviates any gripping you may feel in your hip sockets and knee joints. Also, if your hips are particularly sensitive while stretching in this direction, you can place blocks under your knees for support.

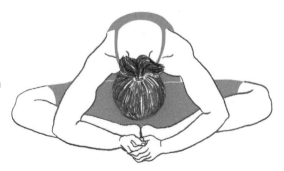

Ananda Balasana Happy Baby Pose

This joyful pose takes place while lying on your back and can be done anywhere, from your yoga mat to your bed. It requires deep hip flexibility, but it can be modified to suit your needs.

Prop: Mat

Precautions: Use caution or avoid this pose if you have recently had a lower-back, knee, hip, hand, or wrist injury or suffer from chronic pain in any of these areas.

Benefits:
- Promotes deep hip flexibility
- Stretches and opens the pelvic floor
- Releases tension and stress

Instructions:

1. Begin by lying flat on top of your yoga mat on your back.

2. Bend both legs and hug them in toward the chest.

3. Take hold of the outer arches of your feet with your hands and bring the bottoms of the feet to face the ceiling.

4. Bring your knees in toward the armpits.

5. Hold for three to five deep breaths.

6. To come out of this pose, slowly release your hands from the feet and bring the legs down.

TIP: If you cannot reach your feet, you can hold on to the hamstrings instead, which are located at the back of the upper legs.

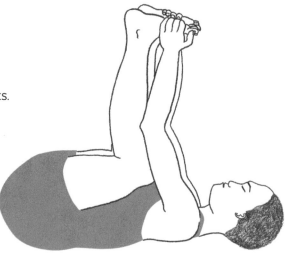

Prasarita Padottanasana I

Wide-Legged Forward Bend

This pose combines the power and stability of a standing pose with the calming nature of a forward fold. It is great for releasing tension from the lower back, hips, and neck, the areas of the body where we hold it most.

Props: Mat, blocks

Precautions: Use caution or avoid this pose if you have recently had a lower-back, knee, hip, hand, wrist, or arm injury or suffer from chronic pain in any of these areas.

Benefits:
- Promotes lower-back flexibility
- Releases tension from the back, hips, and neck
- Calms the body and mind

Instructions:

1. Step into a wide-legged stance, bringing your feet a bit wider than the length of one of your legs.

2. Bring your hands to your hips, bend your knees, send your hips backward, and fold your torso forward and down with a straight spine.

3. Once you are folded over, bring your hands to the floor with your palms flat and elbows pointed back behind you.

4. Allow your head to hang over freely; release control.

5. Hold for three to five breaths.

6. To come out of this pose, press into the floor with both feet and slowly roll up to an upright position.

TIP: If your hands do not reach the floor, you can bend your knees generously or use yoga blocks under your hands to bring the floor to you.

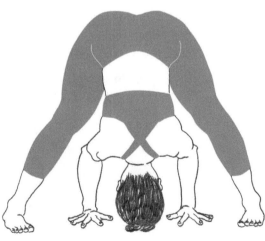

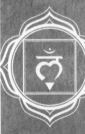

Upavistha Konasana Wide-Angle Pose

This pose provides hip and inner thigh opening, with the calming aspect of a forward fold. It is another great pose for stretching all the key areas of the root chakra, such as the hips and pelvic area.

Props: Mat, blanket

Precautions: Use caution or avoid this pose if you have recently had a lower-back, knee, or hip injury or suffer from chronic pain in any of these areas.

Benefits:
- Opens the hips and inner thighs
- Calms the body and mind

Instructions:

1. Come to a seated position on the floor, sitting up tall on the two sit bones at the base of your pelvis and your legs straight out in front of you.

2. Stretch your legs open to either side and flex your feet, bringing the legs as far open as you can while keeping your knees and toes pointing toward the ceiling.

3. Inhale and lengthen the spine, then exhale and fold the torso forward, stretching the arms out in front of you, looking down.

4. Place your forehead on the floor if you are able to and keep the knees and toes pointed at the ceiling.

5. Hold for three to five breaths.

6. To come out of this pose, on an inhale, gently and slowly walk the hands back in toward the pelvis and bring the torso upright.

7. Bring the legs back in toward the center line of the body.

TIP: Place a folded yoga blanket under your hips and sit on the rounded edge of the blanket to promote a forward tilt of your pelvis. This alleviates any gripping you may feel in your hip sockets and tension in the inner thighs.

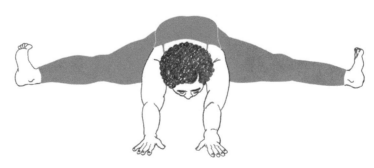

Malasana Garland Pose

This pose is essentially a squat that is helpful for releasing the pelvic floor muscles and gaining flexibility in the hips. It will help release any tension built up in that area.

Props: Mat, block(s)

Precautions: Use caution or avoid this pose if you have recently had a lower-back or knee injury or suffer from chronic pain in either of these areas.

Benefits:
- Hamstring and gluteal muscle stretch
- Promotes hip flexibility
- Relieves stress and tension

Instructions:

1. Stand with your legs and feet externally rotated, toes pointing outward.

2. Bring your feet a bit wider than the distance of your hips and deeply bend both legs, coming into a squat.

3. Bring your hips lower than your knees.

4. Place your hands together to meet at the center of your chest in a prayer position.

5. Hold for three to five deep breaths.

6. To come out of this pose, place your hands on the floor and turn your legs so your feet are parallel to each other while slowly straightening your legs.

7. Bend your knees slightly, bring your hands to your hips, and slowly bring your torso to an upright position.

TIP: If you are not able to fully squat down or if your heels do not touch the floor, try sitting on a yoga block or even a stack of yoga blocks for support. This also alleviates pressure in the hip and knee joints.

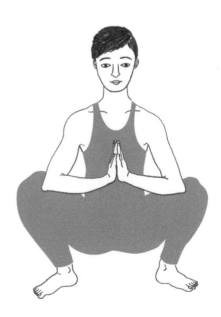

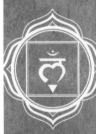

Kapotasana Pigeon Pose

This pose is a bit more complex because it involves deeply stretching the hips in both directions. It also brings the front knee into deep flexion. Pigeon Pose is great for stretching and releasing tension from the hips and pelvic area.

Props: Mat, blanket

Precautions: Use caution or avoid this pose if you have recently had a lower-back, knee, or hip injury or suffer from chronic pain in any of these areas.

Benefits:
- Promotes flexibility in the hips
- Releases tension and stress
- Calms and quiets the mind

Instructions:

1. Begin on your hands and knees, then bring one bent leg forward in between your hands, placing it down on the outer edge of the leg, heel in toward the pubis.

2. Straighten the back leg out behind you, bringing the entire front of that leg and top of that foot to the ground.

3. Inhale and lengthen the spine, then exhale and fold the torso forward. You can either stretch the arms out in front of you or bend the arms and stack the hands on top of each other, palms facing down.

4. Rest your forehead on the floor or on top of your hands.

5. Hold for three to five breaths.

6. To come out of this pose, lift the torso up and place your hands on the floor, using them to press your hips up and step your front leg back so that you return to your hands and knees.

7. Repeat on the other side.

TIP: If your hips do not reach the floor, you can place a folded yoga blanket (or a stack of folded blankets) under your hips for support and to alleviate pressure in the joints. Your front shin does not have to be completely horizonal, and it may be better for your body to keep it on a diagonal.

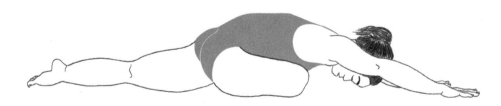

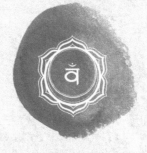

CHAPTER 5

sacral chakra

This chakra is located in the lower abdomen, between the navel and pubis, and it governs our reproductive health and the organs and muscles in the pelvic area. When it is balanced, we experience a healthy sex drive, healthy relationships, and are generally optimistic. Yoga can help balance the sacral chakra by generating a healthy amount of *prana* to that area and releasing any negativity that has built up over time.

Paschimottanasana Seated Forward Bend

This calming, seated forward fold stretches the lower-back and hamstring areas. It will compress and contract the sacral chakra, which is particularly helpful for recovering from trauma in that area.

Props: Mat, blanket

Precautions: Use caution or avoid this pose if you have recently had a lower-back, hamstring, hand, wrist, or arm injury or suffer from chronic pain in any of these areas.

Benefits:
- Promotes hamstring flexibility
- Releases lower-back tension
- Calms the body and mind

Instructions:

1. Begin by sitting up tall on the floor on the two sit bones at the base of your pelvis.

2. Stretch your legs out in front of you and flex your feet, pointing your knees and toes toward the ceiling.

3. Inhale and lengthen the spine, then exhale and fold the torso forward, bringing your hands to your shins, ankles, or feet.

4. Look down toward your legs.

5. Hold for three to five deep breaths.

6. To come out of this pose, gently and slowly bring your torso back to an upright position.

TIP: Place a folded yoga blanket under your hips and sit on the rounded edge of the blanket to promote a forward tilt of your pelvis. This alleviates any gripping you may feel in your hamstrings and lower back.

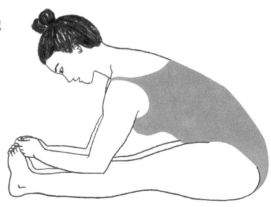

Janu Sirsasana Head-to-Knee Forward Bend

This one-legged forward-bending pose is very relaxing and calming for the body and mind. The sacral chakra is compressed in this pose, as in Seated Forward Bend (page 42), which provides a sense of grounding and security.

Props: Mat, blanket

Precautions: Use caution or avoid this pose if you have recently had a lower-back or hamstring injury or suffer from chronic pain in either of these areas.

Benefits:
- Stretches the hamstrings and lower back
- Relieves tension and stress
- Calms the body and mind

Instructions:

1. Begin by sitting tall on the floor on the two sit bones at the base of your pelvis.

2. Straighten one leg out in front of you, flexing that foot and pointing the knee and toe toward the ceiling.

3. Bend the other leg and turn it out, placing the bottom of that foot to the inner thigh of the straightened leg.

4. Inhale and lengthen the spine, then exhale and fold the torso forward, stretching the arms ahead of you and placing your hands on the floor, framing the straightened leg.

5. Look down and keep as much length in your spine as possible.

6. Hold for three to five breaths.

7. To come out of this pose, on an inhale, slowly and gently bring the torso back upright and straighten the bent leg.

8. Repeat on the other side.

TIP: Place a folded yoga blanket under your hips and sit on the rounded edge of the blanket to promote a forward tilt of your pelvis. This alleviates any gripping you may feel in your hamstrings and lower back.

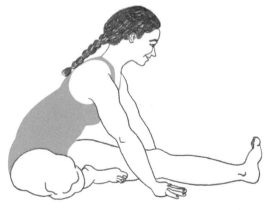

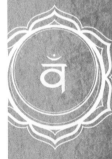

SACRAL CHAKRA

43

Setu Bandha Sarvangasana Bridge Pose

This is an active pose that stretches and opens the hips and pelvic area while working the quadriceps. This will help open and bring light and energy to the sacral chakra while building some heat in that area.

Prop: Mat

Precautions: Use caution or avoid this pose if you have recently had a lower-back, knee, or hip injury or suffer from chronic pain in any of these areas.

Benefits:
- Stretches the quadriceps and the hips
- Strengthens the hamstrings
- Stretches the front of your chest

Instructions:

1. Begin by lying flat on top of your yoga mat on your back.

2. Bend your knees toward the ceiling and bring your feet flat on the floor.

3. Walk the heels in toward the glutes, and bring the feet hip-distance apart and parallel to each other.

4. Press the feet and shoulders into the floor and lift the pelvis up while arching your back.

5. Move your straightened arms toward each other beneath you, roll them to their outer edges, and clasp your hands together under your body.

6. Press your arms into the floor as you gently lift your hips up farther toward the ceiling.

7. Hold for three to five breaths.

8. To come out of this pose, release your hands and gently bring the hips back down to the floor.

TIP: If you are not able to clasp your hands together under your body, you can take hold of the sides of your yoga mat and use your grip to press into the floor and lift your hips up farther.

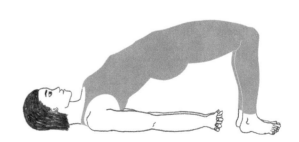

Adho Mukha Svanasana

Downward-Facing Dog Pose

This may be the most famous of the yoga poses, and it's a foundational one that every yogi should know. It is technically an inversion, even though your feet are still planted firmly on the ground. It's great for strengthening the hip flexors to bring some protection and security to the sacral chakra.

Prop: Mat

Precautions: Use caution or avoid this pose if you have recently had a lower-back, knee, hip, hand, or wrist injury or suffer from chronic pain in any of these areas.

Benefits:
- Strengthens the legs, arms, wrists, and hip flexors
- Relaxes the body and mind
- Opens the pelvic floor area

Instructions:

1. Begin on your hands and knees, bringing your hands directly under the shoulders with the palms flat on the floor and the knees directly under the hips.

2. Tuck your toes under and press into the floor with your hands and feet as you straighten the legs and lift the hips, so your legs and back are two diagonal planes rising from the floor.

3. Press your heels toward the floor and continue to lift the hips up and back, away from your hands.

4. Turn the hands out slightly, and keep the arms straight, but do not lock the elbow joints.

5. Relax your head and allow it to hang down.

6. Hold for three to five breaths.

7. To come out of this pose, drop the knees gently onto the floor and return to your hands and knees.

TIP: It is completely fine if your heels do not touch the ground, as long as they are pressing down in that direction energetically. Also, feel free to bend your knees to protect the hamstrings and lower back if they are tight.

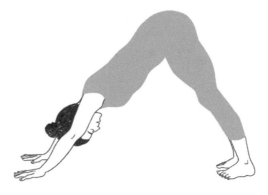

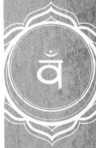

Navasana Boat Pose

This pose is a very challenging abdominal strengthener. It will build muscle and heat in the lower and upper abdominals, bringing comfort and power to the sacral chakra.

Prop: Mat

Precautions: Use caution or avoid this pose if you have recently had an abdominal or hip injury or suffer from chronic pain in either of these areas.

Benefits:

- Strengthens the abdominals, arms, and hip flexors
- Brings power and strength to the abdominal area

Instructions:

1. Begin by sitting on the floor with your legs bent and in front of you.

2. Tilt the torso slightly back and keep your spine straight.

3. Lift the legs up and straighten them one at a time (or both together for more of a challenge), bringing your body into a *V* shape.

4. Reach your arms straight out in front of you, your palms facing each other.

5. Hold for three to five breaths.

6. To come out of this pose, bend the legs and gently bring the legs and arms back down.

TIP: If this pose is too challenging, you can bend your legs and bring the shins parallel to the floor.

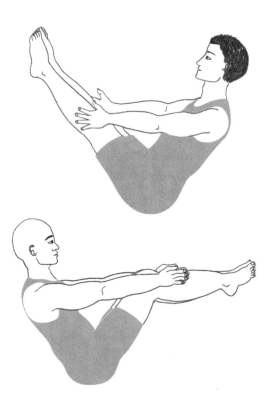

Ashta Chandrasana High Lunge

This is seen as an alternative or preparatory pose for Warrior II Pose, yet it has a great deal of benefits in its own right. This standing pose is a gentle hip opener, a confidence booster, and is very energizing and strengthening for the legs. It will also help energize the sacral chakra and strengthen the muscles in that area.

Prop: Mat

Precautions: Use caution or avoid this pose if you have recently had a lower-back, knee, or hip injury or suffer from chronic pain in any of these areas.

Benefits:
- Strengthens the legs
- Opens the hips and pelvis
- Builds self-confidence

Instructions:

1. Begin in Tadasana (Mountain Pose, page 60) with your feet parallel to each another, hip-distance apart.

2. Step one foot back into a wide stance, approximately the length of one of your legs.

3. Keep the back leg straight with the heel slightly raised.

4. Bend and lunge forward into the front leg, keeping that knee tracking straight above the ankle and in line with the second and third toes.

5. Face forward toward the bent leg with your spine straight.

6. Reach the hands up, palms facing each other, keeping energy in your arms, hands, and fingers while you press your hips down.

7. Hold for three to five breaths.

8. To come out of this pose, bring your hands to your hips and step the back leg up to meet the front leg, returning to Mountain Pose.

9. Repeat on the other side.

TIP: You may need to adjust your stance to accommodate keeping the front knee directly above the ankle. Play around with it and see what works best for you, prioritizing the alignment of the knee over the front bent leg.

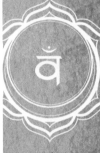

Virabhadrasana II Warrior II Pose

This is one of the most basic and foundational yoga poses, providing the body with strength in the legs and promoting flexibility in the inner thighs and hips. This standing pose will help you feel empowered and bring energy to the sacral chakra.

Prop: Mat

Precautions: Use caution or avoid this pose if you have recently had a lower-back, knee, or hip injury or suffer from chronic pain any of these areas.

Benefits:
- Strengthens the legs
- Opens the hips
- Empowering

Instructions:

1. Begin in a wide-legged stance with your feet about as wide as the distance of one of your legs, your feet parallel to each other.

2. Turn one leg out, facing the toes away from your other foot, and bend that leg.

3. Turn the other leg slightly in, bringing the foot to a 45-degree angle on the floor. Keep this leg straight.

4. Align the heel of the bent leg with the arch of the foot of the straightened leg. Keep your hips on a slight diagonal, turned toward the bent leg.

5. Reach your arms out to either side, your palms facing toward the floor.

6. Turn your head to look over the hand that is out over the bent leg.

7. Hold for three to five breaths.

8. To come out of this pose, slowly and gently straighten the bent leg and bring your hands down to your sides. Bring your legs in toward each other.

9. Repeat on the other side.

TIP: If you find that you are unstable in this pose, engage your abdominal and core muscles while trying to focus your eyes on one single spot. This helps keep you centered and your attention focused to aid your balance.

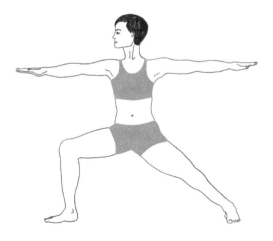

Utkata Konasana Goddess Pose

This is a great active standing pose that will strengthen the legs while promoting external rotation in the hips and opening the pelvis. Goddess Pose will help open and empower the sacral chakra.

Props: Mat; wall, chair, or table

Precautions: Use caution or avoid this pose if you have recently had a lower-back, knee, or hip injury or suffer from chronic pain in any of these areas.

Benefits:
- Promotes hip opening
- Empowering

Instructions:

1. Begin in a wide-legged stance, bringing your feet about as wide as the length of one of your legs.

2. Turn the legs and feet out from the hips so that your toes are facing away from one another.

3. Bend your legs, bringing your upper thighs parallel to the floor in a wide-legged squatting position.

4. Reach your arms out to the sides and bend your elbows, palms facing forward.

5. Look slightly up and hold your gaze there.

6. Hold for three to five breaths.

7. To come out of this pose, slowly and gently straighten the legs and bring the arms down. Bring your feet in toward each other.

TIP: You do not have to bring the upper thighs all the way down to a parallel position to the floor if you are not able to, especially if you are feeling pressure in the knees. You can also hold on to a wall, table, or the back of a chair with one or both hands if you would like some extra support, as this can be a very active and energetic pose.

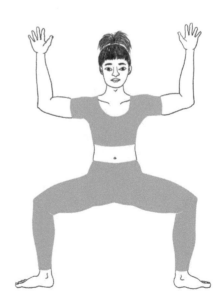

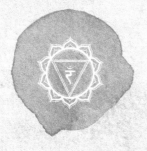

CHAPTER 6

solar plexus chakra

This chakra is located at the center of the abdominal area, above the navel and below the chest, and it governs our self-confidence and self-control. When this area is balanced, we will have a strong sense of self and believe that we can do anything. Yoga can help balance this chakra with poses that open the area and build a sense of inner confidence.

Marjaryasana Cat Pose

This is a great pose to counter the back-bending poses, as it stretches the back in the opposite direction. This pose is typically done flowing from Cow Pose (page 52) and the combination of the two warms up the entire body from the spine outward. This encloses, presses, and protects the solar plexus chakra and provides a sense of security in the area.

Prop: Mat

Precautions: Use caution or avoid this pose if you have recently had a back, knee, hand, or wrist injury or suffer from chronic pain in any of these areas.

Benefits:
- Stretches the upper back
- Calming and soothing
- Quiets the mind

Instructions:

1. Begin on your hands and knees, bringing the hands directly under the shoulders with the palms flat on the floor and the knees directly under the hips. Your spine should be straight and flat.

2. On an exhale, curve the spine, reaching the upper back toward the ceiling and hanging the head down, looking behind you from beneath your body.

3. Hold for the whole exhale and release on the inhale, either to a flat back or straight into Cow Pose.

4. Repeat Cat Pose, or the sequence of Cat Pose to Cow Pose, for eight to ten repetitions.

TIP: If your knees are sensitive on the floor, you can fold and double up your yoga mat to provide extra cushion, or use a small folded blanket.

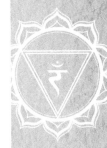

Bitilasana Cow Pose

This is the partner pose to Cat Pose (page 51) as the two are often practiced together in coordinated movement and breath. This pose is done on the inhale, opening the chest and heart center and providing a stretch to the solar plexus chakra.

Prop: Mat

Precautions: Use caution or avoid this pose if you have recently had a back, knee, hip, hand, or wrist injury or suffer from chronic pain in any of these areas.

Benefits:
- Opens the chest and heart center
- Energizes the body

Instructions:

1. Begin on your hands and knees, bringing the hands directly under the shoulders with the palms flat on the floor and the knees directly under the hips. Your spine should be straight and flat.

2. On an inhale, arch the back, looking up, spreading the shoulders apart and reaching the heart center forward.

3. Hold for the whole inhale and release on the exhale, either into a flat back or straight into Cat Pose.

4. Repeat Cow Pose, or the sequence of Cow Pose to Cat Pose, for eight to ten repetitions.

TIP: Avoid locking into your elbow joints, as this could cause injury to the area. Hold yourself up using your arm muscles instead, and if you have a tendency to hyperextend the elbows, practice using a microbend instead of keeping the arms completely straight.

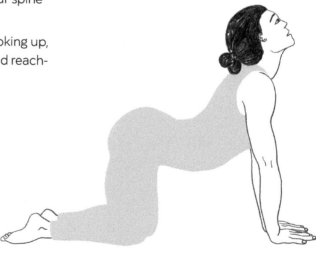

Ardha Matsyendrasana

Half Lord of the Fishes Pose

This is a seated twist that provides a combination of hip flexibility and torso twisting. It also aids in spinal movement and mobility, bringing a level of protection and comfort to the solar plexus chakra.

Prop: Mat

Precautions: Use caution or avoid this pose if you have recently had a back, knee, or hip injury or suffer from chronic pain in any of these areas.

Benefits:
- Promotes hip flexibility
- Promotes spinal health and mobility
- Relaxing and calming

Instructions:

1. Come to a seated position on the floor with your legs stretched out in front of you.

2. Bend your right leg and cross it over your left leg, the right foot flat on the floor and the knee pointed up to the ceiling.

3. Bend the left leg in, bringing the heel toward the right glute.

4. Reach your left arm toward the floor, wrapping it around the upper portion of the right leg. Bring your right arm behind you and place it on the floor, palm down.

5. Inhale and lengthen the spine, exhale and gently twist the upper body toward the top leg.

6. As you sit in the twist, continue to lengthen the spine on the inhale and twist a bit deeper on the exhale.

7. Hold for three to five breaths.

8. To come out of this pose, gently unwind from the twist and uncross the legs.

9. Repeat on the other side.

TIP: If you are not able to keep both hips on the floor in this pose, try stretching the bottom leg straight out in front of you instead of bending it.

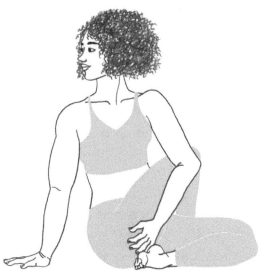

Utthita Trikonasana Extended Triangle Pose

This standing pose is very empowering and strengthening for the legs. It will provide a sense of confidence and power to the solar plexus area while energizing the body.

Props: Mat, block

Precautions: Use caution or avoid this pose if you have recently had a back, knee, hip, hand, or wrist injury or suffer from chronic pain in any of these areas.

Benefits:
- Strengthens the legs
- Stretches the inner thighs
- Empowering

Instructions:

1. Begin in a wide-legged stance with your feet about as wide as the length of one of your legs, your feet parallel to each other.

2. Turn one leg out, facing the toes away from your other foot, and keep both legs straight.

3. Turn the opposite leg slightly in, bringing the foot to a 45-degree angle on the floor.

4. Align the heel of the front leg with the arch of the back foot. Your hips should be on a slight diagonal and turned toward the front leg.

5. Reach your arms straight out to either side and face your palms toward the floor.

6. Reach your torso over the front leg until you cannot reach any farther out, then place your front hand on your shin, ankle, foot, or the floor.

7. Press down into that hand and, with your shoulders straight, reach your other arm straight up toward the ceiling as you direct your gaze upward.

8. Hold for three to five breaths.

9. To come out of this pose, press into the floor with your feet and use your abdominals to lift your torso upright.

10. Repeat on the other side.

TIP: You can place your supporting hand on a yoga block instead of your leg or the floor. You can also place your hand behind the foot on the floor or on a block to get more of a shoulder and chest opening.

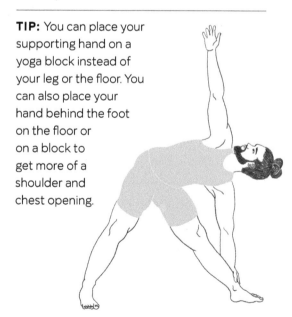

Bhujangasana Cobra Pose

This arch is a great stretch for the front of the torso, including your chest and abdominal area. It is active, but not as active as many of the other deep back-bending poses, and it will help open and stretch the solar plexus chakra area.

Prop: Mat

Precautions: Use caution or avoid this pose if you have recently had a back, knee, hip, hand, or wrist injury or suffer from chronic pain in any of these areas.

Benefits:
- Strengthens the arms
- Stretches the front of the body
- Provides energy and power

Instructions:

1. Begin by lying flat on top of your yoga mat on your belly.

2. Bend your arms so your hands are flat on the floor under your shoulders and your elbows point up to the ceiling.

3. Place your forehead on the floor.

4. On an inhale, press into the floor with your hands, lifting your entire torso off the floor, arching your back.

5. Make sure your arms are shoulder-width apart and straight.

6. Keep your energy moving up toward the ceiling through the crown of your head and press your hips gently into the floor.

7. Hold for three to five breaths.

8. To come out of this pose, slowly and gently release your torso down to the floor, bringing your forehead back to the ground.

TIP: You can work your way up to this pose by practicing Low Cobra Pose (page 61), a smaller backbend that is detailed in chapter 7.

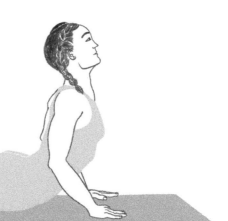

Urdhva Mukha Svanasana

Upward-Facing Dog Pose

This is a more energetic alternative to Cobra Pose (page 55) as your legs are lifted off the floor and you use your arms to hold you up. It is strengthening for the arms and back, while it also stretches the front of your body. This will help open the solar plexus chakra area.

Prop: Mat

Precautions: Use caution or avoid this pose if you have recently had a back, knee, hip, hand, or wrist injury or suffer from chronic pain in any of these areas.

Benefits:

- Strengthens the arms
- Stretches the front of the body
- Provides energy and power

Instructions:

1. Begin by lying flat on top of your yoga mat on your belly.

2. Bend your arms so your hands are flat on the floor under your shoulders and your elbows point up to the ceiling.

3. Place your forehead and the tops of your feet flush against the floor.

4. On an inhale, press into the floor with your hands, lift your entire torso off the floor, arch your back, and lift the fronts of your legs off the floor, resting your weight on your hands and the tops of your feet.

5. Hold this pose while looking up, keeping length in your neck and your shoulders away from the ears.

6. Hold for three to five breaths.

7. To come out of this pose, press into the floor with your hands, lift your hips up and back, tuck the toes under, and come into Downward-Facing Dog Pose (page 45).

TIP: If this pose is too challenging, you can substitute it with Cobra Pose (page 55) or Low Cobra Pose (page 61). You can work up to the full expression of this pose as you build arm strength.

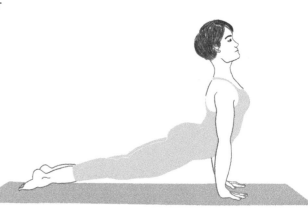

Dhanurasana Bow Pose

This deep back-bending pose opens the front of the body and presses the abdominal area into the ground. It provides a sense of grounding as well as an opening to the solar plexus area.

Props: Mat, strap

Precautions: Use caution or avoid this pose if you have recently had a back, neck, shoulder, arm, or wrist injury or suffer from chronic pain in any of these areas.

Benefits:
- Opens the front of your body
- Very energizing
- Grounding

Instructions:

1. Begin by lying flat on top of your yoga mat on your belly.

2. Bend both legs up toward your head and take hold of the outer arches of both feet with your hands.

3. Inhale and lift the head and feet up toward the ceiling, forming a *U* shape with your body.

4. Reach your head and feet up toward the ceiling while bringing your heart center forward.

5. Hold for three to five breaths.

6. To come out of this pose, gently bring your head and legs back down to the floor and release your hands from your feet.

TIP: If this pose is too much for you, you can begin by stretching one leg at a time, using one hand or even using a strap if you cannot reach your foot with your hand. You can work your way toward practicing the full expression of the pose.

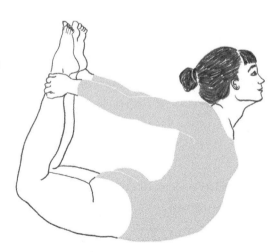

Natarajasana Dancer Pose

This pose is an advanced backbend and balancing pose. It combines back flexibility, hip flexibility, and balance. If it is too challenging, you can work toward the full expression of this pose over time with training. This is another opener for the solar plexus chakra area.

Prop: Mat

Precautions: Use caution or avoid this pose if you have recently had a lower-back, knee, hip, hand, or wrist injury or suffer from chronic pain in any of these areas.

Benefits:
- Stretches the back
- Opens the front of the body
- Gains balance and stability

Instructions:

1. Begin by standing tall in Mountain Pose (page 60) with your feet parallel to each other.

2. Bend the right leg and take hold of the foot in your right hand, holding the inner arch of the foot behind you.

3. Lift the right foot and leg up, deeply arching your back and balancing on the left leg.

4. Reach your left arm out in front of you, palm up.

5. Continue reaching the right foot up toward the ceiling.

6. Hold for three to five breaths.

7. To come out of this pose, slowly and gently bring the leg down and release the hand from the foot.

8. Repeat on the other side.

TIP: You can use a yoga strap to hold the foot behind you if you cannot reach the foot with your hand. Wrap the looped strap around the top of your foot and hold on to the ends of the strap with both of your hands raised behind your head.

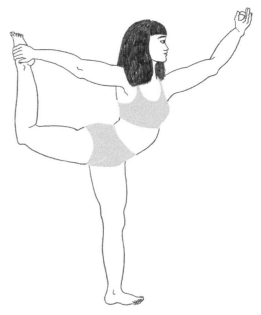

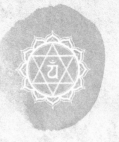

CHAPTER 7

heart chakra

This chakra is located at the heart center, and it governs our ability to love ourselves and others unconditionally as well as trust and forgive. A balanced heart chakra will allow us to fully accept and give love to others. Yoga can help balance the heart chakra by using heart-opening poses that bring the heart center forward.

Tadasana Mountain Pose (Variation with Hands Clasped)

While Mountain Pose is often thought of as a simple yoga pose, it requires a great deal of energy and attention to detail. The simplicity of Mountain Pose combined with this energetic chest opener is great for unblocking and healing the heart chakra. It creates grounding and stability in the body, and the arching of the back allows energy to flow more freely to the heart chakra.

Prop: Mat

Precautions: Use caution or avoid this pose if you have recently had an upper-back, arm, hand, or wrist injury or suffer from chronic pain in any of these areas.

Benefits:
- Heart opening
- Promotes back flexibility
- Energizing

Instructions:

1. Stand at the top of your yoga mat with your feet either hip-distance apart or with your big toes together and heels about an inch apart.

2. Interlock your fingers behind you, at the small of your back, and reach your hands down toward your heels.

3. Look up, arch your back, and reach your heart center forward and up.

4. Hold for three to five breaths.

5. To come out of this pose, on an inhale, release your back from the arch, bring your hands back up to the small of your back, and release your hands from the clasp.

TIP: If this chest opening is too deep, you can hold on to a strap instead, bringing the hands wider apart and opening the chest and heart less.

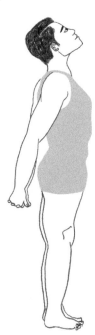

Ardha Bhujangasana Low Cobra Pose

This pose is an alternative or precursor to Cobra Pose (page 55). It is a great upper-back strengthener and perfect for opening the heart center while gently arching the back.

Prop: Mat

Precautions: Use caution or avoid this pose if you have recently had an upper-back or neck injury or suffer from chronic pain in either of these areas.

Benefits:
- Strengthens the upper back
- Energizing
- Opens the heart

Instructions:

1. Begin by lying flat on top of your yoga mat on your belly.

2. Bend your arms so your hands are on the floor under your shoulders and your elbows point up to the ceiling.

3. Place your forehead on the floor.

4. On an inhale, lift your head and chest off the floor, coming into a small upper-back arch and keeping your elbows bent.

5. Use your upper-back muscles to lift and hold you up.

6. Hold for an inhale, and lower back down on an exhale.

7. Repeat three to five times.

TIP: Practice using your upper-back muscles to hold you up by slightly hovering your hands above the floor.

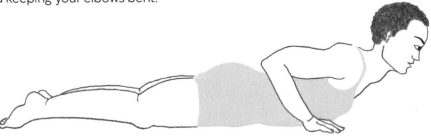

Salamba Bhujangasana

Sphinx or Supported Cobra Pose

While this pose may look simple, it is actually very active, as you are constantly pressing the chest forward between the hands. However, it is a bit less active than other backbends, as you are moving into a smaller upper-back arch. It's excellent for opening the heart chakra area.

Prop: Mat

Precautions: Use caution or avoid this pose if you have recently had an upper-back, arm, or elbow injury or suffer from chronic pain in any of these areas.

Benefits:
- Promotes back flexibility
- Opens the heart
- Energizing

Instructions:

1. Begin by lying flat on top of your yoga mat on your belly.

2. Bend your arms so your hands are on the floor under your shoulders and your elbows point up to the ceiling.

3. Place your forehead on the floor.

4. On an inhale, lift your head and chest up and bring your forearms in front of you, parallel to each other, with your hands flat on the floor and fingertips pointed away from you.

5. Hold yourself up by pressing your forearms into the floor and actively reaching your chest forward.

6. Hold for three to five breaths.

7. To come out of this pose, slowly and gently come off your elbows, bring your arms to your sides, and place your forehead on the floor.

TIP: If your elbows feel uncomfortable on the floor, you can fold your yoga mat for extra cushion.

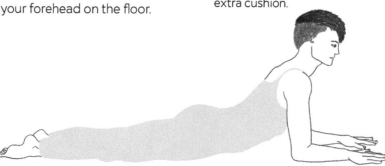

Anahatasana Melting Heart Pose

This stretch is also known as Puppy Pose and is often seen in yin yoga. Because you stretch forward with your head down, it's great for helping open the heart chakra while calming the body and mind.

Prop: Mat

Precautions: Use caution or avoid this pose if you have recently had a back or knee injury or suffer from chronic pain in either of these areas.

Benefits:
- Promotes back flexibility
- Calms and soothes the mind
- Opens the heart

Instructions:

1. Begin on your hands and knees, bringing the hands directly under the shoulders with the palms flat on the floor and the knees directly under the hips. Your shins should be parallel on the floor behind you.

2. Slide your hands forward, straightening the arms, and bring the forehead to the floor.

3. Reach the heart center down to the floor and open the armpits.

4. Hold for three to five breaths.

5. To come out of this pose, gently lift the head upright, walk the hands back toward the legs, and come to sitting upright.

TIP: You can double up your yoga mat to provide cushion under the knees, or use a folded yoga blanket under the head as well.

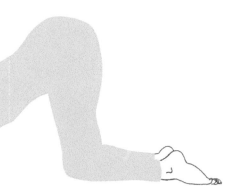

Camatkarasana Wild Thing

This is a very fun, energizing, and creative pose that stretches the front of the body. In reaching up to the sky with your heart center, you open the heart chakra to prepare for giving and receiving love.

Prop: Mat

Precautions: Use caution or avoid this pose if you have recently had a back, hamstring, hip, hand, wrist, or arm injury or suffer from chronic pain in any of these areas.

Benefits:

- Opens the heart
- Strengthens the arms and legs
- Promotes back flexibility

Instructions:

1. Begin in Downward-Facing Dog Pose (page 45).

2. Lift the right leg up behind you and turn it out from the hip.

3. Bring the right foot across the back body and to the floor behind you, turning the front of your body to face the ceiling.

4. Straighten the left leg out and keep the left hand on the floor.

5. Reach the right arm back and arch your back. Reach and stretch!

6. Hold for three to five breaths.

7. To come out of this pose, shift your weight fully back onto the left leg, lean into the left hand on the floor, and turn the body back around to face the floor, placing the right hand and right foot down and leveling the hips to return to Downward-Facing Dog Pose.

8. Repeat on the other side.

TIP: You can use your breath while holding this pose to increase and deepen your arch just a bit each time you exhale.

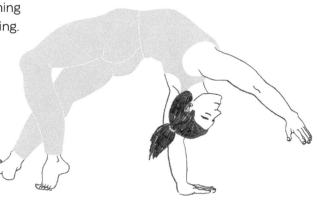

Matsyasana Fish Pose

This energizing backbend will help open and release tension from the area surrounding the heart chakra.

Prop: Mat

Precautions: Use caution or avoid this pose if you have recently had a back, arm, or elbow injury or suffer from chronic pain in any of these areas.

Benefits:
- Promotes back flexibility
- Opens the heart
- Energizing

Instructions:

1. Begin by lying flat on top of your yoga mat on your back with your legs straight out and feet flexed.

2. Reach the heart and chest up toward the ceiling and bend your elbows, propping yourself up with the elbows on the floor.

3. Tip your head back and place the top of your head on the floor and look behind you.

4. Hold for three to five breaths.

5. To come out of this pose, slowly and gently bring your elbows out from under your upper body and release the back of your head down to the floor, releasing your body from the arch.

TIP: Be mindful of keeping energy in your feet and legs during this pose. You can flex them or point them forward for a different kind of stretch in the tops of your feet.

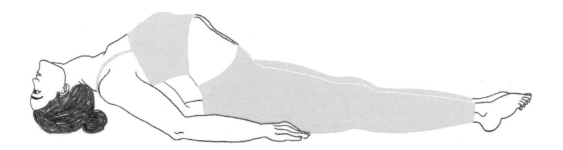

Ustrasana Camel Pose

This deep backbend provides plenty of heart-opening benefits for the heart chakra. It is energizing and stretches the entire front body, including the chest, abdominal area, and quadriceps.

Props: Mat, blocks

Precautions: Use caution or avoid this pose if you have recently had a back, knee, hip, hand, wrist, or arm injury or suffer from chronic pain in any of these areas.

Benefits:
- Opens the heart and chest
- Promotes back flexibility
- Energizing

Instructions:

1. Stand on your knees, bringing them hip-distance apart with your shins parallel to each other behind you.

2. Tuck your toes under, flexing the feet.

3. Cup your hands on your heels behind you, arms turned slightly outward, and reach your heart and chest forward. Your head should be tilted back to face the ceiling.

4. Hold for three to five breaths.

5. To come out of this pose, gently and slowly engage the abdominals and remove your hands from your heels, coming back to standing on the knees.

TIP: Instead of bringing your hands all the way to your heels, an alternative is to place your hands on top of yoga blocks placed at any height at the outer edges of the feet. This can help you work your way up to eventually placing the hands to the feet.

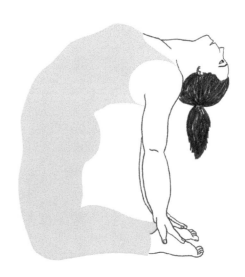

Urdhva Dhanurasana

Upward-Facing Bow or Wheel Pose

This is an advanced back-bending pose that you can work up to if it is too challenging. A deep backbend, it also provides opening and stretching in the front of the body. It will help open the heart and provide more energy to that area.

Props: Mat, strap

Precautions: Use caution or avoid this pose if you have recently had a back, knee, neck, shoulder, arm, or wrist injury or suffer from chronic pain in any of these areas.

Benefits:
- Promotes deep back flexibility
- Opens the front of your body
- Very energizing

Instructions:

1. Begin by lying flat on top of your yoga mat on your back.

2. Bring your feet flat on the floor, hip-distance apart, and point your knees up toward the ceiling.

3. Rotate your arms up and behind you, placing your hands on either sides of your ears on the floor with your fingertips pointing toward your shoulders and elbows pointing up to the ceiling.

4. Press into the floor with your hands and feet and lift your hips up, bringing your body into a wide upside-down *U* shape, keeping your hands shoulder-width apart and legs hip-distance apart.

5. Press your hips up toward the ceiling energetically as you continue to press your hands and feet into the floor.

CONTINUED »

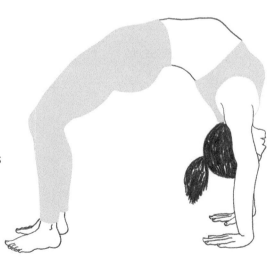

Urdhva Dhanurasana CONTINUED

6. Allow your head to hang down between your arms.

7. Hold for three to five breaths.

8. To come out of this pose, slowly and gently release your body down onto the mat while tucking your chin to your chest.

9. Engage the abdominal muscles for a few breaths and then hug the legs in toward the chest.

TIP: A great alternative is Bridge Pose (page 44). You can practice Bridge Pose to work your way up to Upward-Facing Bow if it's feeling too advanced. Once you are able to practice Upward-Facing Bow, you can help keep your arms shoulders-distance apart by using a yoga strap placed around the upper arms.

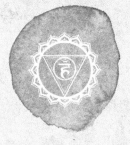

CHAPTER 8

throat chakra

This chakra is located at the throat in the neck area, and it governs our ability to speak up for ourselves and what we believe in. When this chakra is balanced, we are able to communicate and express ourselves clearly with our unique voices or through other methods, such as writing. Yoga can help bring balance to the throat chakra by stretching and releasing the muscles in the neck while opening up the area.

Assisted Neck Stretches in Sukhasana

Easy Pose

This is a great stretch for all the muscles around the neck. We tend to carry quite a bit of stress and tension in the neck, so it is very beneficial to stretch that area. This exercise provides release and relaxation for the throat chakra.

Prop: Mat

Precautions: Use caution or avoid this pose if you have recently had an upper-back or neck injury or suffer from chronic pain in either of these areas.

Benefits:
- Promotes flexibility and mobility in the neck
- Reduces neck-muscle tension
- Relaxes the body and mind

Instructions:

1. Come into Easy Pose by sitting on the floor in a cross-legged position, with your shins crossed in front of your body and your feet flexed beneath the knees. Sit up tall on the two sit bones at the bottom of the pelvis.

2. To stretch the back of the neck, tilt the head forward and gently hold on to the top of the head with your fingertips, stretching it forward and down.

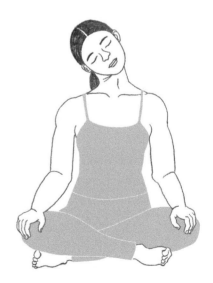

3. To stretch the front of the neck, look up, keeping the rest of your body stable.

4. To stretch the sides of the neck, tilt the head to the right, holding on to the top of the head with the right hand, and gently pull it toward your right shoulder. Repeat on the left side.

5. Hold each stretch for three to five breaths before lifting the head to an upright position.

TIP: Place a folded yoga blanket under your hips and sit on the rounded edge of the blanket to promote a forward tilt of your pelvis. This alleviates any gripping you may feel in your hip sockets and knee joints.

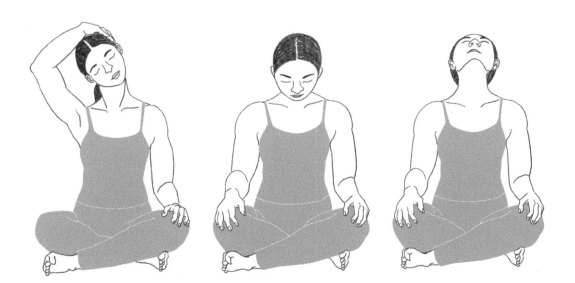

Neck Rolls in Sukhasana Easy Pose

This series of continually flowing movements will help you release tension in the muscles all around the neck, providing a release for the throat chakra and surrounding areas.

Prop: Mat

Precautions: Use caution or avoid this pose if you have recently had an upper-back or neck injury or suffer from chronic pain in either of these areas.

Benefits:

- Stretches the neck
- Mobilizes the neck and shoulders
- Relaxes and quiets the mind

Instructions:

1. Come into Easy Pose by sitting on the floor in a cross-legged position with your shins crossed in front of your body and your feet flexed under the knees. Sit up tall on the two sit bones at the bottom of the pelvis.

2. Bring your hands, palms down, to your knees.

3. While keeping your body still, tuck your chin to your chest and begin to rotate the head around in one direction slowly, smoothly, and continually for eight to ten repetitions.

4. Repeat on the other side.

TIP: Try to avoid rotating the head around too quickly, as it can cause injury. The key to these neck rolls is slow and smooth movements. Do not forget to breathe!

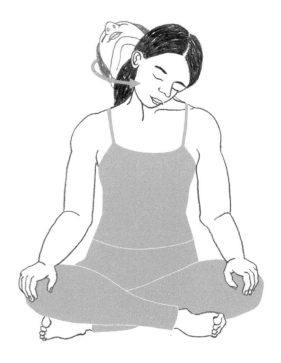

Sukhasana with Jalandhara Bandha

Easy Pose with Chin Lock

This relaxing pose is practiced with one of the *bandhas* (see page 25). It is very simple but effective in creating a calming, protective, and supportive environment for the throat chakra. It is perfect for healing after experiencing trauma in the area.

Props: Mat, blanket

Precautions: Use caution or avoid this pose if you have recently had an upper-back or neck injury or suffer from chronic pain in either of these areas.

Benefits:
- Calms, soothes, and quiets the mind
- Stretches the back of the neck
- Hips, glutes, and hamstring stretch

Instructions:

1. Come into Easy Pose by sitting on the floor in a cross-legged position, with your shins crossed in front of the body and your feet flexed under the knees. Sit up tall on the two sit bones at the bottom of the pelvis.

2. Bring your hands, palms down, to your knees.

3. Tuck your chin to your chest and bring your chest up to meet your chin halfway.

4. Remain here for three to five breaths.

5. To come out of this pose, gently lift the head back upright.

TIP: Place a folded yoga blanket under your hips and sit on the rounded edge of the blanket to promote a forward tilt of your pelvis. This alleviates any gripping you may feel in your hip sockets and knee joints.

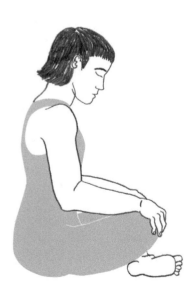

Salamba Matsyasana Supported Fish Pose

This is a much less active and more restorative version of Fish Pose (page 65) but will provide a very different energy and feeling. It is great for opening and releasing the throat chakra.

Props: Mat, blocks, blanket

Precautions: Use caution or avoid this pose if you have recently had an upper-back or neck injury or suffer from chronic pain in either of these areas.

Benefits:
- Relaxing and restorative
- Opens the chest, heart, and throat area

Instructions:

1. Begin by aligning your yoga blocks on your mat: one where your head will go at the block's medium height, and one at the block's lowest height where your mid-back will be.

2. Lie down on top of your yoga blocks. Adjust your yoga blocks if necessary so the one beneath your back is horizontal at the bottom edge of your shoulder blades. The other block should be beneath the back of your head, where it can remain comfortably for several minutes.

3. Once your blocks are settled and you are comfortable, place your hands by your sides, palms facing up, and stretch your legs straight out in front of you.

4. Rest for several minutes, closing your eyes and focusing your attention on your breathing.

5. To come out of this pose, engage your abdominal muscles and add slight and gentle motion back into your limbs.

6. Bend your legs and roll off the yoga blocks to the right side of the body. Rest there for a few deep breaths before making your way up to a seated upright position.

TIP: An alternative to using yoga blocks is a rolled-up yoga blanket. Roll your blanket into a long, skinny roll and place it along the spine, from under your head to the upper- to mid-back.

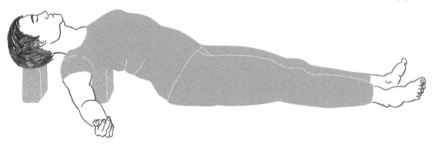

Ashtangasana Knees, Chest, Chin Pose

This pose is often used in sun salutations as an alternative to Four-Limbed Staff Pose (page 83). It is a great chest, neck, and throat opener and will help open the throat chakra.

Prop: Mat

Precautions: Use caution or avoid this pose if you have recently had an upper-back, arm, hand, or wrist injury or suffer from chronic pain in any of these areas.

Benefits:
- Chest, heart, and throat opener
- Energizing

Instructions:

1. Begin by lying flat on top of your yoga mat on your belly with your forehead down, hands flat on the floor under your shoulders, and elbows pointing up to the ceiling.

2. Tuck your toes and flex your feet, and bend your knees but keep them on the floor.

3. Press into the floor with your hands and look forward, bringing your back into an arch while allowing your chin and chest to rest on the floor.

4. Your knees, chest, chin, and hands should all be on the floor. Most of your weight is being held by your hands.

5. Hold for three to five breaths.

6. To come out of this pose, gently look toward the floor, straighten your legs, and bring your hips and abdomen back to the floor.

TIP: If you are feeling pain in your chin and neck area, it is likely that you are placing too much weight there. Try holding yourself up a bit more with your hands instead to alleviate some of the pressure.

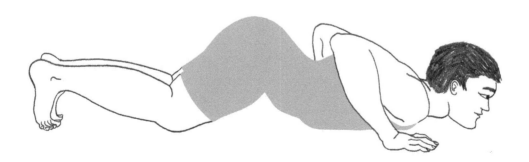

Uttanasana Standing Forward Bend

This is a very simple yet relaxing pose that provides a sense of calm while stretching the lower back, hamstrings, and glutes. It allows the head and neck to relax and release tension, providing calm and release for the throat chakra.

Props: Mat, blocks

Precautions: Use caution or avoid this pose if you have recently had a back, neck, hip, knee, or leg injury or suffer from chronic pain in any of these areas.

Benefits:
- Calming and relaxing
- Promotes hamstring and hip flexibility
- Reduces neck tension

Instructions:

1. Stand at the top of your yoga mat with your feet parallel to each other and hip-distance apart.

2. Bring your hands to your hips and fold your torso over with a straight spine.

3. Release your hands to the floor and allow your head to relax and hang over.

4. Hold for three to five breaths.

5. To come out of this pose, bring your hands to your hips, slightly bend your knees, and roll your torso back upright to standing.

TIP: If your hands do not reach the floor, you can place yoga blocks under them at any height that works for you. You can also bend your knees generously. Avoid letting the hands dangle or hang.

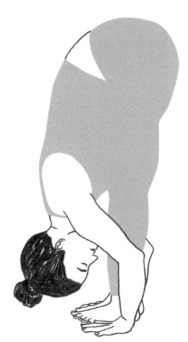

Halasana Plow Pose

This is a forward fold literally flipped upside down. You are performing the same action of folding forward, except your back and neck are on the floor instead of your legs. This pose will provide your throat chakra a sense of protection and security.

Props: Mat, blanket

Precautions: Use caution or avoid this pose if you have recently had an upper-back, arm, hand, or wrist injury or suffer from chronic pain in any of these areas.

Benefits:
- Calms and soothes the mind and body
- Stretches the back
- Promotes hamstring flexibility

Instructions:

1. Begin by lying flat on top of your yoga mat on your back with your arms at your sides.

2. Press into the floor with your hands and lift your legs and hips up and over your head, bringing your feet onto the floor behind your head.

3. Keep your hands pressing flat into the floor behind your back and straighten your legs.

4. Your chin should be tucked into the chest.

5. Hold for three to five breaths.

6. To come out of this pose, bend the legs and gently and slowly release the back onto the floor.

TIP: This is often practiced as a precursor to Supported Shoulder Stand (page 78), which uses a yoga blanket placed under the upper back. The yoga blanket will give you a bit more space between your cervical spine (the back of the neck) and the floor. Using a yoga blanket is a much safer variation of Plow Pose and should be used especially if going directly into Supported Shoulder Stand.

Salamba Sarvangasana

Supported Shoulder Stand

Often practiced right after Plow Pose (page 77), this pose is one of the most calming inversions of the yoga asanas. Similar to Plow Pose, this pose will provide the throat chakra with a sense of protection, safety, and comfort.

Props: Mat, blanket

Precautions: Use caution or avoid this pose if you have recently had a back, neck, arm, hand, or wrist injury or suffer from chronic pain in any of these areas.

Benefits:
- Promotes blood flow to the upper body
- Calming and soothing
- Quiets the mind

Instructions:

1. Come into Plow Pose (page 77).

2. Lift one leg at a time up toward the ceiling, keeping the feet pointed but the toes flexed. (This is sometimes referred to as Barbie Foot—picture how a Barbie doll's foot is positioned and replicate it.)

3. Place your hands flat on your upper back and keep the elbows tucked in toward each other. Do not turn your head while in Supported Shoulder Stand. This could cause neck injury.

4. Hold for three to five breaths—or more, depending on your ability.

5. To come out of this pose, slowly lower one foot at a time back through Plow Pose, and then gently bring your back down to the floor, following with the legs.

TIP: If your back is not used to this pose, it can cause a bit of a shock to those muscles, especially if you hold this pose for a longer period of time. To avoid spasming, activate the abdominal muscles after coming out of this pose, which support the back.

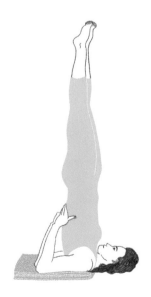

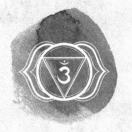

CHAPTER 9

third-eye chakra

This chakra is located at the center of the forehead between the eyebrows. It governs concentration and focus within the mind, and it allows us to have healthy and clear thoughts. When this chakra is balanced, we will be able to concentrate on tasks easily and achieve what we set our minds to. Yoga can help balance this chakra by activating, grounding, and energizing the area, allowing us to center in on our third eye and observe what is happening there.

Balasana Child's Pose

This is a simple and basic pose that is very relaxing, thanks to its forward-folding nature. Since your forehead is physically touching the floor in this pose, it is grounding and calming for the third-eye chakra. It is great for centering yourself and connecting your mind with your body.

Props: Mat, blanket

Precautions: Use caution or avoid this pose if you have recently had a knee, hip, or back injury or suffer from chronic pain in any of these areas.

Benefits:
- Promotes hip flexibility
- Cooling and calming
- Relaxing for the body and mind

Instructions:

1. Begin on your hands and knees and touch your big toes together behind you.

2. Separate your knees and relax your torso over your thighs, bringing your forehead to the floor.

3. Stretch your arms out in front of you, palms facing down.

4. Relax here for three to five breaths.

5. To come out of this pose, gently move upright to a seated position.

TIP: If you are not able to sit comfortably on your heels in this pose, you can take a folded yoga blanket and place it on top of your calves. Then you can sit your hips onto the blanket, or on multiple blankets, so you can relax.

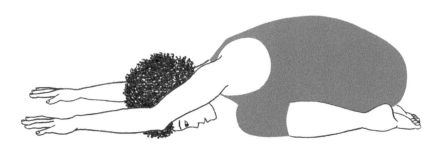

Prone Savasana Prone Corpse Pose

There is a well-known version of this pose called Savasana (Corpse Pose, page 93), which is practiced lying on the back. This version is practiced in the opposite direction by lying on your belly. Because the center of the forehead is planted down, this pose is very calming, grounding, and centering for the third-eye chakra.

Props: Mat, blanket

Precautions: Use caution or avoid this pose if you have recently had a neck or hand injury or suffer from chronic pain in either of these areas.

Benefits:
- Very calming and relaxing
- Aids insomnia and restlessness

Instructions:

1. Begin by lying flat on top of your yoga mat on your belly.

2. Bend your arms and stack one hand on top of the other below your head, then place your forehead on the back of your top hand.

3. Keep your legs straight behind you and relax them completely.

4. Hold for three to ten minutes.

5. Halfway through your time in this pose, lift your head slightly off your hands and bring the other hand on top. Then place your head back down and continue with the remaining time you have allowed for yourself (equal to the time you spent with your forehead on the opposite hand).

6. To come out of this pose, lift your head off your hands and bring your hands under your shoulders, palms flat on the floor.

7. Using your hands, press yourself up onto your hands and knees and come to a seated position.

TIP: If you are having trouble resting your feet on the floor, you can roll up a blanket and place it under your ankles, where they can rest comfortably. You can go into this pose with your hands by your sides, palms facing up, turning your head to one side and resting on your cheek. If you choose this option, it is not as grounding for the third-eye chakra, but it is still calming. Be sure to switch to turn your head to the other side halfway through to maintain symmetry in the body.

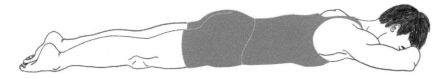

Kumbhakasana Plank Pose

This pose is more familiar than you think! It is actually the same pose you use for a push-up. It is also a full-body workout all on its own, and it is quite challenging to hold for long periods of time. This pose is very engaging and activating for the third-eye chakra because there is a lot of energy flowing outward through the head.

Prop: Mat

Precautions: Use caution or avoid this pose if you have recently had an arm, back, or leg injury or suffer from chronic pain in any of these areas.

Benefits:
- Strength building
- Full-body workout
- Energizing

Instructions:

1. Begin on your hands and knees, bringing your hands directly under the shoulders with the palms flat on the floor and the knees hip-distance apart.

2. Step one foot back at a time, coming onto the balls of your feet, bringing the legs straight out behind you.

3. Keep the body in one straight line from the top of your head, down your entire spine and down the legs, all the way to your heels.

4. Hold the pose and keep the body activated for three to five breaths.

5. To come out of this pose, lower the knees down to the floor one at a time and take the weight off your hands, coming to a seated position.

TIP: If this pose is too challenging, you can place your knees on the floor, keeping the upper legs at a diagonal with the upper body. This will take some of the pressure off your arms, making it a bit easier to hold. Practice this way until you feel strong and comfortable enough to bring your knees off the ground.

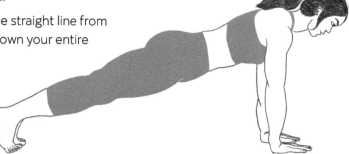

Chaturanga Dandasana Four-Limbed Staff Pose

This is otherwise known as a half push-up because you are lowering the body only halfway down. In many ways, this can be more challenging than a normal push-up because it requires more strength to hold yourself in that position without going all the way down to the floor. This pose is grounding for the third-eye chakra because it sends energy from that chakra downward, toward the earth, activating it.

Prop: Mat

Precautions: Use caution or avoid this pose if you have recently had a neck, back, or arm injury or suffer from chronic pain in any of these areas.

Benefits:
- Strengthens the arms and shoulders
- Builds focus and concentration
- Energizing

Instructions:

1. Begin on your hands and knees, bringing your hands directly under the shoulders with the palms flat on the floor and the knees hip-distance apart.

2. Step one foot back at a time, coming onto the balls of your feet, your legs straight out behind you.

3. Keep the body in one straight line from the top of your head, down your entire spine and down the legs, all the way to your heels.

4. Hold the pose and keep the body activated for three to five breaths.

5. Keeping the body in one straight line, lower yourself halfway down, bringing the arms to about a 90-degree angle.

6. Avoid lowering the shoulders below the elbows, as this could cause injury.

7. To come out of this pose, press your hands into the floor and shift your body into Upward-Facing Dog Pose (page 56).

TIP: An alternative to this pose is Knees, Chest, Chin Pose (page 75). It is a bit easier on the arms because you are also bearing some of your weight on the chest and chin.

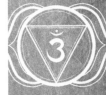

Viparita Karani Legs Up the Wall Pose

This is a very calming and relaxing restorative pose. It can be done if you have been standing on your feet all day, or even after you've been traveling on an airplane or otherwise sitting, to relieve swelling in your legs and ankles. It helps calm the third-eye chakra and open your mind to new possibilities in your life.

Props: Mat, blanket, wall, strap

Precautions: Use caution or avoid this pose if you have recently had a back, hip, or leg injury or suffer from chronic pain in any of these areas.

Benefits:
- Calming and restorative
- Opens the mind
- Relaxes the body

Instructions:

1. Place a folded blanket at the base of a wall, with the rounded edge positioned one or two inches away from it.

2. Scoot your glutes and sit bones up to the wall's edge and lie on your right side with your knees bent.

3. Roll onto the top of the folded blanket, with your lower back on the blanket and your feet on the wall.

4. Straighten your legs up the wall, resting the backs of your legs against it.

5. Relax your feet and keep your legs hip-distance apart.

6. Place your hands on the floor by your sides, palms up, and close your eyes.

7. Hold for one to five minutes.

8. To come out of this pose, bend both legs, bringing the bottoms of your feet to the wall.

9. Roll onto the right side of your body and rest there for a few deep breaths before coming back upright.

TIP: If you find that your legs are falling out to the sides while you are resting in this pose, try looping a yoga strap around your shins to keep the legs hip-distance apart.

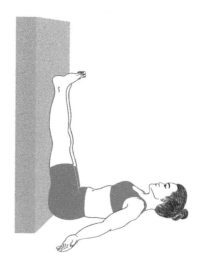

Baddha Konasana Variation Butterfly Pose

This pose is a variation on Bound-Angle Pose (page 35) with the addition of a forward fold and a yoga block to hold the head up. The variation is from the yin yoga technique. This pose is very grounding for the third-eye chakra because the forehead is placed on top of a yoga block.

Props: Mat, block

Precautions: Use caution or avoid this pose if you have recently had a neck or back injury or suffer from chronic pain in either of these areas.

Benefits:
- Promotes hip flexibility
- Grounding
- Relaxing

Instructions:

1. To begin, come into Bound-Angle Pose (page 35).

2. With the bottoms of the feet together, bring the heels in toward the pelvis, about 12 inches away or closer, depending on your proportions.

3. Place the yoga block in its highest position in the diamond-shaped space between your legs, closer to your heels than your pelvis.

4. Come to a forward fold, placing your forehead on top of the yoga block.

5. You may need to adjust your feet and the placement of the block to find a comfortable spot in your forward fold. Just make sure your spine is as lengthened as possible.

CONTINUED ››

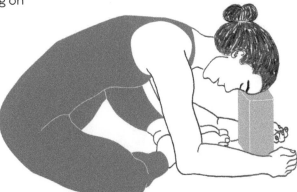

6. Place your hands on either sides of your feet on the floor with the palms facing up.

7. Hold for one to five minutes, depending on your personal ability or as instructed, if you are practicing this pose as part of a sequence.

8. To come out of this pose, lift your head off the block and come up to a seated upright position.

TIP: You can treat this pose as a meditation, since it is held a bit longer than the others. As you relax here, close your eyes and deepen your breath. Focus on your inhales and exhales for as long as you are able to, and if a thought comes into your mind, gently set it to the side and come back to focusing on the breath. Repeat that step as many times as needed while you are holding the pose.

Gomukhasana Cow Face Pose

This pose is a deep-hip opener and can be challenging for yoga beginners. You do not have to strive to stack the knees directly on top of each other, as shown in the illustration, if your body does not allow you to do so. Be kind to your body and do not force it into this or any yoga pose. The third-eye chakra is activated here, as you are engaging in a great amount of concentration and focus.

Props: Mat, strap

Precautions: Use caution or avoid this pose if you have recently had a knee, hip, neck, shoulder, or arm injury or suffer from chronic pain in any of these areas.

Benefits:
- Promotes hip and shoulder flexibility
- Releases tension and stress

Instructions:

1. To begin, come to a seated position on the floor, sitting up tall on your sit bones.

2. Turn the legs out from the hips and bend both legs.

3. Bring the right heel in toward the left glute and rest the outer right thigh on the floor.

4. Cross your left leg on top of the right leg, and bring the left heel in toward the right glute.

5. Bring your knees as close to alignment with each other in the center line of your body as possible without forcing it.

6. Raise your right arm and bend it behind your head with your fingertips between your shoulder blades. Lower your left arm and bend it up, bringing the hand to the upper back.

CONTINUED »

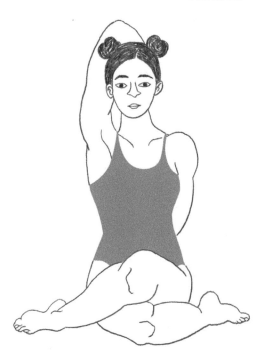

7. Hook the fingers of both hands together, holding your hands at your upper back.

8. Point your right elbow up and your left elbow down. Sit up tall, lengthening the spine as you face forward.

9. Hold for three to five breaths.

10. To come out of this pose, release your hands and bring the arms down. Uncross your legs, and repeat on the other side.

TIP: If you find that you are not able to hook your fingertips together and hold your hands behind your back, you can drape a strap over one shoulder and hold on to the strap with your hands at your upper back instead.

Adho Mukha Vrksasana Handstand

This is an advanced inversion, but beginner and intermediate yoga students can use a wall to help practice this pose. Once you build your strength and get used to being upside down on your hands, you can work toward moving away from the wall. This is activating and grounding for the third-eye chakra because as you hold the pose, your energy flows down from that chakra into the floor.

Props: Mat, wall

Precautions: Use caution or avoid this pose if you have recently had a back, neck, arm, or leg injury or suffer from chronic pain in any of these areas.

Benefits:
- Strengthens the arms
- Promotes balance
- Shifts your perspective

Instructions:

1. Come to a clear wall space and bring your fingertips about one handprint away from the wall's edge.

2. Bring the hands shoulders-distance apart and come into Downward-Facing Dog Pose (page 45). Your back should be facing the wall.

CONTINUED »

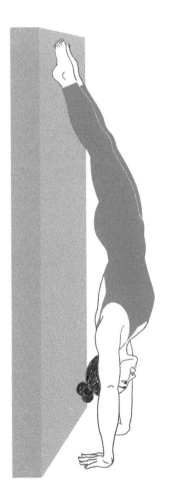

3. Step the right foot up and back over your body toward the wall, then kick the left leg up back toward the wall, gently propelling the hips to stack above your shoulders.

4. Rest the heels of both feet on the wall above you, keeping your legs straight and feet flexed.

5. You should be looking down at the floor between your hands the entire time, neck straight.

6. Hold for three to five breaths.

7. To come out of this pose, engage the core and abdominal muscles and release one foot from the wall to gently set it down on the floor. The other leg will follow.

8. Step both feet back into Downward-Facing Dog Pose.

9. Lower the knees to the floor and sit the hips back into Child's Pose (page 80). You can rest there for as long as needed before repeating on the other side (kicking the left foot up to the wall first).

TIP: If you feel comfortable being upside down in Handstand and would like to try it without the assistance of the wall, you can still practice by the wall, but bring your feet a few inches away from it once you are up in the pose to test your balance. Continually reach the heels toward the ceiling and press the hands down toward the floor to help you stabilize. Come back to resting the heels on the wall when needed.

CHAPTER 10

crown chakra

This chakra is located just above the top of the head, and it governs our ability to connect with a higher source and our purpose. If this chakra is balanced, we will have a clear idea of our direction in life, and what we are meant to do. We will also feel a strong connection with the higher power that is guiding our life in its intended direction. Yoga can help balance this chakra by connecting our energy to this area and directing it in a precise and focused way, allowing us to observe what is happening right now.

Tadasana Mountain Pose

This is the most important foundational yoga pose because it is where your alignment should always refer back to in each and every pose. This pose helps activate and initiate the crown chakra by the nature of its simplicity and by directing energy upward, through the top of the head.

Prop: Mat

Precautions: Use caution or avoid this pose if you have recently had a knee, hip, or leg injury or suffer from chronic pain in any of these areas.

Benefits:
- Grounding
- Centering
- A great place to begin

Instructions:

1. Stand up tall on both feet, bringing your big toes to touch and separating your heels one to two inches apart.

2. Place your arms at your sides, palms facing the body.

3. Look forward and focus your eyes on one spot.

4. Stand here for three to five breaths.

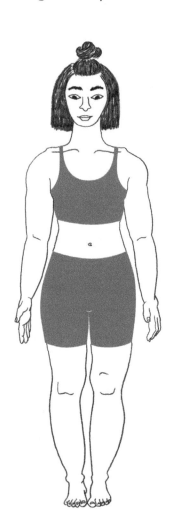

TIP: If you are feeling unstable in this pose with your feet together, a great alternative is to keep your feet parallel and hip-distance apart. This creates a wider base for more stability in the body.

Savasana Corpse Pose

This is the pose that is often done at the end of a yoga practice. It helps you quiet the mind and relax the body. This allows you to connect to your crown chakra by drawing your attention inward and observing how you feel inside.

Props: Mat, blanket

Precautions: Use caution or avoid this pose if you have recently had a knee, hip-joint, or lower-back injury or suffer from chronic pain in any of these areas.

Benefits:
- Promotes relaxation
- A great pose to practice meditation
- Grounding and centering

Instructions:

1. Begin by lying flat on top of your yoga mat on your back.

2. Separate your legs slightly and relax them completely.

3. Place your arms at your sides and turn your palms up toward the ceiling.

4. Close your eyes and begin to deepen your inhales.

5. Focus on the inhales and exhales.

6. Relax here, focusing on the breath, for three to ten minutes, depending on your personal ability, or as instructed if you're practicing this pose as part of a sequence.

7. To come out of this pose, first allow slight and gentle motion back into the body, then bend the legs and roll to rest on the right side of the body, with your legs bent and your right arm under your head.

8. When you are ready, make your way up to a seated position.

TIP: There are many variations to Savasana. To ease any lower-back pain you may be feeling by lying flat on the floor, place a rolled yoga blanket under the knees.

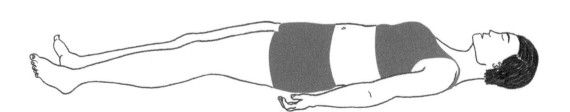

Vrksasana Tree Pose

This is a wonderful balancing pose that helps center the mind and body. It is a great strengthener for the core and legs. Reaching energy up and out through the top of the head in this pose helps initiate and activate the crown chakra.

Prop: Mat

Precautions: Use caution or avoid this pose if you have recently had a knee, hip, or foot injury or suffer from chronic pain in any of these areas.

Benefits:
- Promotes balance
- Strengthens the core

Instructions:

1. To begin, stand up tall, bringing your feet parallel, then raise your right leg and turn it out from the hip.

2. Place the bottom of your right foot on your left inner thigh. Avoid placing the foot on the knee joint.

3. Bring your hands to meet at the center of your chest in prayer position. For more of a challenge with your balance, you can raise your arms above your head with your palms facing each other.

4. Hold for three to five breaths.

5. To come out of this pose, release your foot back to the floor and bring your arms down.

6. Repeat on the other side.

TIP: If your foot does not reach the upper inner thigh, you can place the foot on the lower leg and shin area instead.

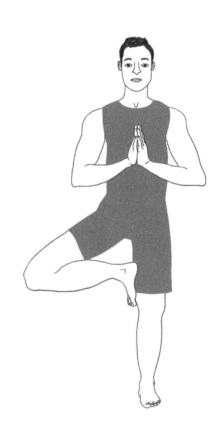

Anjaneyasana Variation Crescent Lunge with Arms Up

This is another variation of High Lunge (page 47). This version is very energizing and activates the crown chakra. As you reach the arms up and come into a slight arch, you are energizing the body and channeling that energy up and out through the top of your head.

Prop: Mat

Precautions: Use caution or avoid this pose if you have recently had a knee or hip-joint injury or suffer from chronic pain in either of these areas.

Benefits:
- Promotes energy
- Strengthens the lower body

Instructions:

1. Come into High Lunge (page 47).

2. Raise the arms up above the head, palms facing each other.

3. Bring your upper back into a slight arch while looking up and reaching the heart center up.

4. Hold for three to five breaths.

5. To come out of this pose, release your back from the arch and return to standing.

6. Repeat on the other side.

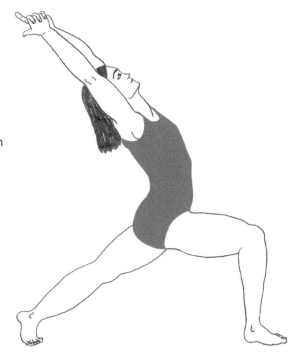

Vasisthasana Side Plank Pose

This energizing pose strengthens your arms and sides. It's great for the crown chakra, activating and centering the mind as you reach energy outward on a diagonal plane through the top of your head.

Prop: Mat

Precautions: Use caution or avoid this pose if you have recently had an arm, wrist, hand, or leg injury or suffer from chronic pain any of these areas.

Benefits:

- Strengthens the obliques and arms
- Very energizing

Instructions:

1. Come into Plank Pose (page 82).

2. Turn onto your left hand, lifting the right hand off the floor and keeping your body in a straight, diagonal line, and stack the right leg and foot on top of the left.

3. Reach the right arm toward the ceiling and turn your head to look up at it.

4. Hold for three to five breaths.

5. To come out of this pose, turn to face the floor and bring your right hand and foot back into Plank Pose.

6. Repeat on the other side for symmetry.

TIP: You can place the bottom knee on the floor if you are feeling unstable or need to first build up arm strength to hold this pose.

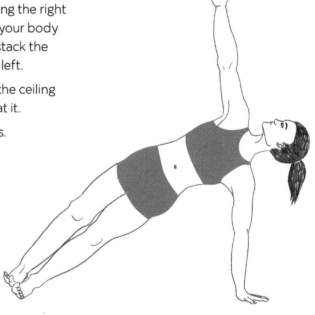

Utthita Parsvakonasana

Extended Side-Angle Pose

This standing pose is a great leg strengthener and requires a bit of flexibility in the hips. The diagonal reach of the arm and head activates the heart chakra.

Props: Mat, block

Precautions: Use caution or avoid this pose if you have recently had a knee, hip, back, leg, or arm injury or suffer from chronic pain in any of these areas.

Benefits:
- Strengthens the legs
- Promotes hip flexibility
- Energizing

Instructions:

1. Come into Warrior II Pose (page 48) with the right foot forward.

2. Reach down to place your right hand or fingertips on the floor outside the right foot.

3. Reach your left arm up and over your left ear, palm down. Continue reaching that left hand and your head out and up in a continual diagonal line.

4. Look up toward the ceiling.

5. Hold for three to five breaths.

6. To come out of this pose, press into the ground with your feet and lift your torso back upright through Warrior II Pose.

7. Repeat on the other side to maintain symmetry in the body.

TIP: You can place your hand on a yoga block set at any height instead of on the floor to create more space in the hip joint of your bent leg.

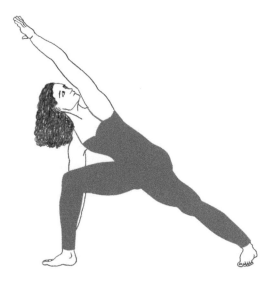

Ardha Chandrasana Half-Moon Pose

This is a challenging balancing pose that requires strength, concentration, and focus. While you are in this pose, direct energy outward through the top of your head, where the crown chakra is located. This helps you balance and activates the crown chakra.

Props: Mat, block

Precautions: Use caution or avoid this pose if you have recently had a knee, hip, back, leg, or arm injury or suffer from chronic pain in any of these areas.

Benefits:
- Strengthens the legs
- Helps improve your balance
- Energizing

Instructions:

1. Come into Extended Triangle Pose (page 54) with the right foot forward.

2. Shift your weight onto your right leg, lifting the left leg until it is parallel to the floor. Flex the left foot and keep it straight and parallel to the floor.

3. Place your right hand on the floor, about 12 inches away from your right foot, or more or less depending on your proportions. Reach your left arm straight up toward the ceiling.

4. Look down at the floor, or straight ahead, or up to the ceiling if your balance enables you to do so.

5. Hold for three to five breaths.

6. To come out of this pose, bend the right leg and gently place the left foot on the floor, and then stand.

7. Repeat on the other side for symmetry in the body.

TIP: You can place your hand on a yoga block instead of the floor to find more length in your spine in this pose.

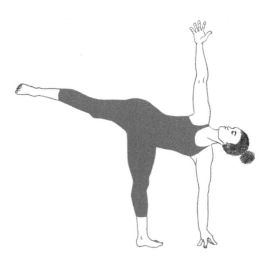

Salamba Sirsasana Supported Headstand

This yoga inversion helps the crown chakra, since placing your head on the floor allows you to send energy through this chakra into the earth. Placing the top of your head on the floor is also quite calming, while the inverted positioning of the body is energizing.

Props: Mat, blanket

Precautions: Use caution or avoid this pose if you have recently had a neck, back, or arm injury or suffer from chronic pain in any of these areas.

Benefits:
- Calms the body and mind
- Changes your perspective

Instructions:

1. Place a blanket, folded into a square shape, at the edge of a wall.

2. Come to Child's Pose (page 80) at the wall, with your elbows and hands on the blanket.

3. Clasp your hands together, then open your hands while keeping your fingers linked. Bring the backs of your hands to face the wall.

4. Place the top of your head on the blanket between your hands, rolling the back of your head into your open palms.

CONTINUED »

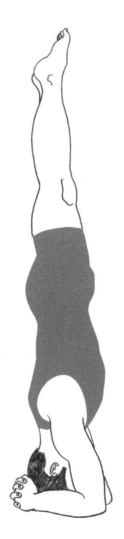

5. Straighten your legs and knees off the floor, and bring your hips up to stack above your shoulders, and your shoulders to stack above your neck and head.

6. Gently place your feet on the wall behind you and straighten your legs to rest your heels on the wall.

7. Hold for three to five breaths.

8. To come out of this pose, bend both legs and gently bring one foot at a time back down to the floor.

9. Sit back into Child's Pose for a few deep breaths and come upright when you are ready.

TIP: If you feel comfortable being upside down in Headstand and would like to try it away from the wall, you can still practice by the wall, but bring your feet a few inches away from it to test your balance once you are up in the pose. Continually reach the heels toward the ceiling and press the hands into the floor to keep you balanced and return to resting the heels on the wall when needed.

CHAPTER 11

healing multiple chakras

We can heal and unblock more than one chakra through our yoga practice, since every yoga pose and sequence is unique and multifaceted. The sequence of the poses together also activates, balances, and heals more than one chakra at once. This makes the possibilities of healing the chakras endless. The yoga sequences that follow offer a glimpse of what can be achieved during a journey through chakra yoga.

Activating and Grounding the Midsection

This yoga sequence activates and grounds the midsection of your body, where the root, sacral, solar plexus, and heart chakras live. Your exploratory journey into these four chakras will allow you to learn more about them within yourself, while also balancing their energies.

Props: Mat, blanket, block

Precautions: Use caution or avoid this sequence if you have recently had a knee, hip, back, leg, or arm injury or suffer from chronic pain in any of these areas.

Benefits:

- Balances the root chakra, sacral chakra, solar plexus chakra, and heart chakra
- A great beginner yoga routine
- A perfect place to start your journey

Poses:

A. Balasana (Child's Pose, page 80)

B. Marjaryasana (Cat Pose, page 51)

C. Bitilasana (Cow Pose, page 52)

D. Ardha Bhujangasana (Low Cobra Pose, page 61)

E. Bhujangasana (Cobra Pose, page 55)

F. Adho Mukha Svanasana (Downward-Facing Dog Pose, page 45)

G. Virabhadrasana (Warrior II Pose, page 48)

H. Utthita Trikonasana (Extended Triangle Pose, page 54)

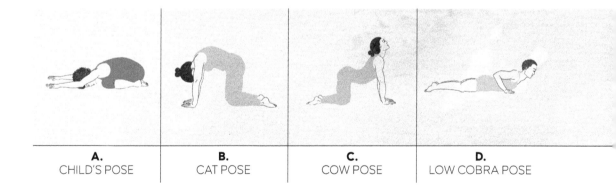

| **A.** CHILD'S POSE | **B.** CAT POSE | **C.** COW POSE | **D.** LOW COBRA POSE |

I. Janu Sirsasana (Head-to-Knee Forward Bend, page 43)

J. Baddha Konasana (Bound-Angle Pose, page 35)

K. Ananda Balasana (Happy Baby Pose, page 36)

L. Savasana (Corpse Pose, page 93)

Instructions:

1. Come into **Child's Pose** and hold for three to five breaths.

2. Come up through your hands and knees and move through **Cat** and **Cow Poses**, breathing in on the **Cow Pose** and out on the **Cat Pose**.

3. Lower yourself down onto your belly and lift the chest and head into **Low Cobra Pose**. Repeat **Low Cobra** three times and hold each pose for one breath.

4. Press up into **Cobra Pose**.

5. Sit back into **Child's Pose**.

6. Press into the floor with your hands, lift your hips slightly, tuck your toes, and straighten your legs into **Downward-Facing Dog Pose**.

7. Step your right foot forward in between your hands, coming into **Warrior II Pose** on the right side.

8. Straighten the right leg and move straight into **Extended Triangle Pose** on the right side.

CONTINUED »

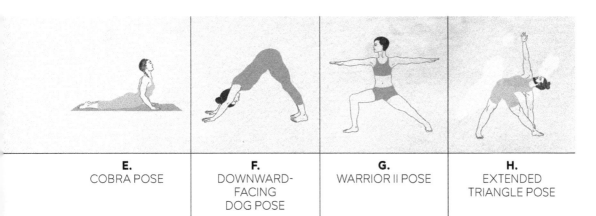

| **E.** COBRA POSE | **F.** DOWNWARD-FACING DOG POSE | **G.** WARRIOR II POSE | **H.** EXTENDED TRIANGLE POSE |

9. Come back into **Downward-Facing Dog Pose** and repeat **Warrior II Pose** on the left side.

10. Straighten the left leg and come straight into **Extended Triangle Pose** on the left side.

11. Come back through **Downward-Facing Dog Pose**, then place the knees on the floor and sit.

12. Stretch the left leg out, coming into **Head-to-Knee Pose** on the right. Hold for three to five breaths.

13. Bend the left leg and come into **Bound-Angle Pose**. Hold for three to five breaths.

14. Straighten the right leg and come into **Head-to-Knee Pose** on the left. Hold for three to five breaths.

15. Lie flat on your back and bring your legs up into **Happy Baby Pose**. Hold for three to five breaths.

16. Straighten the legs out onto the floor into **Savasana** and remain there for three to ten minutes.

TIP: Feel free to use the yoga props wherever needed, and do not feel ashamed about using them. Even the most advanced yoga practitioners still use yoga props to maintain proper alignment in the body and to avoid injury.

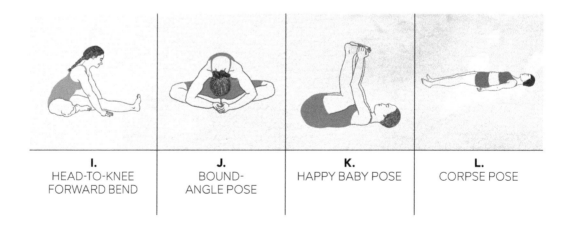

| **I.** HEAD-TO-KNEE FORWARD BEND | **J.** BOUND-ANGLE POSE | **K.** HAPPY BABY POSE | **L.** CORPSE POSE |

Drawing Attention and Focus to the Upper Chakras

This yoga sequence focuses on the upper chakras, allowing you to observe what is happening in those areas. This is a great way to begin your journey in exploring the upper chakras, as they are often the most difficult ones for us to connect to.

Props: Mat, blanket block

Precautions: Use caution or avoid this sequence if you have recently had a knee, hip, back, leg, or arm injury or suffer from chronic pain in any of these areas.

Benefits:
- Balances the throat chakra, third-eye chakra, and crown chakra

Poses:

A. Assisted Neck Stretches in Sukhasana: Easy Pose (page 70)

B. Balasana (Child's Pose, page 80)

C. Kumbhakasana (Plank Pose, page 82)

D. Vasisthasana (Side Plank Pose, page 96)

E. Ashtangasana (Knees, Chest, Chin Pose, page 75)

F. Urdhva Mukha Svanasana (Upward-Facing Dog Pose, page 56)

CONTINUED ››

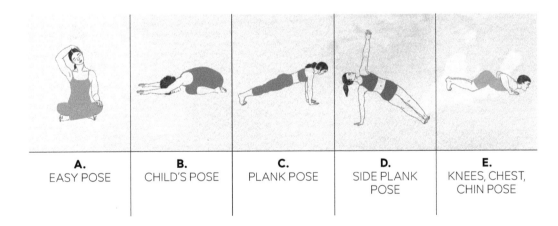

| A. EASY POSE | B. CHILD'S POSE | C. PLANK POSE | D. SIDE PLANK POSE | E. KNEES, CHEST, CHIN POSE |

G. Adho Mukha Svanasana (Downward-Facing Dog Pose, page 45)

H. Ashta Chandrasana (High Lunge with arms up, page 47)

I. Vrksasana (Tree Pose, page 94)

J. Salamba Sirsasana (Supported Headstand, page 99)

K. Halasana (Plow Pose, page 77)

L. Salamba Sarvangasana (Supported Shoulder Stand, page 78)

M. Savasana (Corpse Pose, page 93)

Instructions:

1. Begin by sitting on the floor in **Easy Pose** and practicing the **Assisted Neck Stretches**.

2. Then move onto your hands and knees and into **Child's Pose**.

3. Come into **Plank Pose**.

4. Shift into **Side Plank Pose** on the right side.

5. Then do **Side Plank Pose** on the left side.

6. Come back through center and move into **Knees, Chest, Chin Pose**.

7. Press into **Upward-Facing Dog Pose**.

8. Shift into **Downward-Facing Dog Pose**.

9. Step the right foot into **High Lunge** with arms up on the right side.

10. Bring the left leg forward to meet the right leg and come into **Tree Pose** on the left side.

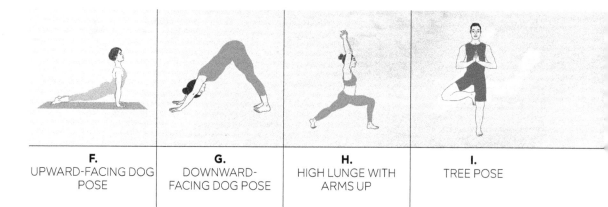

| **F.** UPWARD-FACING DOG POSE | **G.** DOWNWARD-FACING DOG POSE | **H.** HIGH LUNGE WITH ARMS UP | **I.** TREE POSE |

11. Step the left foot back through **High Lunge** with arms up and come back into **Downward-Facing Dog Pose**.

12. Step the left foot forward into **High Lunge** with arms up on the left.

13. Bring the right leg up into **Tree Pose** on the right side.

14. Step the right leg back through **High Lunge** with arms up and into **Downward-Facing Dog Pose**.

15. Move to a wall and come into **Supported Headstand**.

16. Come out of your headstand and away from the wall, moving into **Plow Pose**.

17. Then lift your legs up into **Supported Shoulder Stand**.

18. Come out of **Supported Shoulder Stand** and engage your abdominal muscles for several deep breaths.

19. Relax into **Savasana** for three to ten minutes.

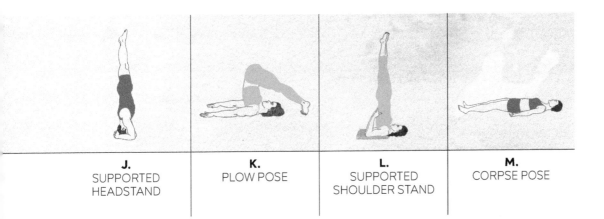

J.
SUPPORTED
HEADSTAND

K.
PLOW POSE

L.
SUPPORTED
SHOULDER STAND

M.
CORPSE POSE

Paying Attention to the Extremities

While this sequence focuses on several chakras, it mainly allows you to activate your arms and legs, or the extremities that these chakras control. Use this sequence if you are feeling a bit anxious and in need of some quiet grounding.

Props: Mat, blanket, block

Precautions: Use caution or avoid this sequence if you have recently had a knee, hip, back, leg, or arm injury or suffer from chronic pain in any of these areas.

Benefits:
- Balances the root chakra, sacral chakra, heart chakra, throat chakra, and third-eye chakra

Poses:

A. Sukhasana with Jalandhara Banda (Easy Pose with Chin Lock, page 73)

B. Navasana (Boat Pose, page 46)

C. Tadasana (Mountain Pose with hands clasped behind, page 60)

D. Uttanasana (Standing Forward Bend, page 76)

E. Tadasana (Mountain Pose with arms at sides, page 92)

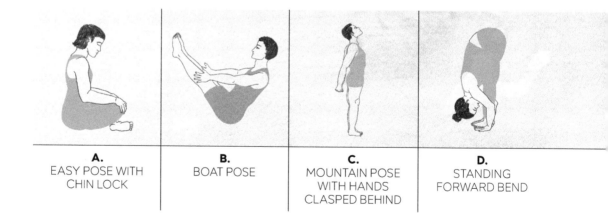

| **A.** EASY POSE WITH CHIN LOCK | **B.** BOAT POSE | **C.** MOUNTAIN POSE WITH HANDS CLASPED BEHIND | **D.** STANDING FORWARD BEND |

F. Prasarita Padottanasana I (Wide-Legged Forward Bend, page 37)

G. Utkata Konasana (Goddess Pose, page 49)

H. Utthita Parsvakonasana (Extended Side-Angle Pose, page 97)

I. Ardha Chandrasana (Half-Moon Pose, page 98)

J. Gomukhasana (Cow Face Pose, page 87)

K. Viparita Karani (Legs Up the Wall Pose, page 84)

Instructions:

1. Come into **Easy Pose with Chin Lock** and hold for several deep breaths.

2. Shift into **Boat Pose**.

3. Come up to standing and move into **Mountain Pose** with your hands clasped behind you.

4. Come into **Standing Forward Bend**.

5. Stand back up into **Mountain Pose** with arms at sides.

CONTINUED »

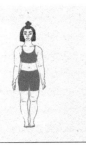

E.
MOUNTAIN POSE
WITH ARMS AT
SIDES

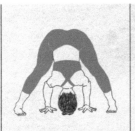

F.
WIDE-LEGGED
FORWARD BEND

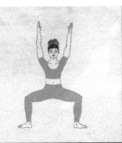

G.
GODDESS POSE

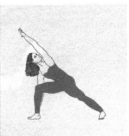

H.
EXTENDED SIDE-
ANGLE POSE

6. Step your legs into **Wide-Legged Forward Bend**.

7. Stand up and come into **Goddess Pose**.

8. Move into **Extended Side-Angle Pose** on the right.

9. Move straight into **Half-Moon Pose** on the right.

10. Come through **Extended Side-Angle Pose** on the left, stand up, and go into **Side-Angle Pose** on the left.

11. Move into **Half-Moon Pose** on the left.

12. Sit down and make your way into **Cow Face Pose** on the right.

13. Come into **Cow Face Pose** on the left.

14. Make your way to a wall and come into **Legs Up the Wall Pose**.

15. Relax there for three to ten minutes.

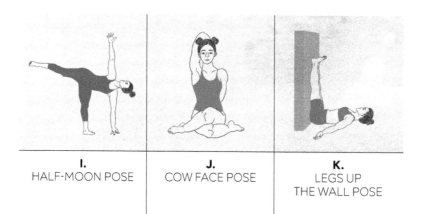

| **I.** HALF-MOON POSE | **J.** COW FACE POSE | **K.** LEGS UP THE WALL POSE |

Building a Strong Foundation

This is a great sequence if you are looking to start from the ground up. Beginning with a strong foundation is good for balancing the chakras in the entire body. Begin from the root and work your way up!

Props: Mat, blanket, block

Precautions: Use caution or avoid this sequence if you have recently had a knee, hip, back, leg, or arm injury or suffer from chronic pain in any of these areas.

Benefits:
- Balancing the root chakra, sacral chakra, and solar plexus chakra

Poses:

A. Siddhasana (Accomplished Pose, page 33)

B. Paschimottanasana (Seated Forward Bend, page 42)

C. Janu Sirsasana (Head-to-Knee Forward Bend, page 43)

D. Ardha Matsyendrasana (Half Lord of the Fishes Pose, page 53)

E. Marjaryasana (Cat Pose, page 51)

F. Bitilasana (Cow Pose, page 52)

CONTINUED ››

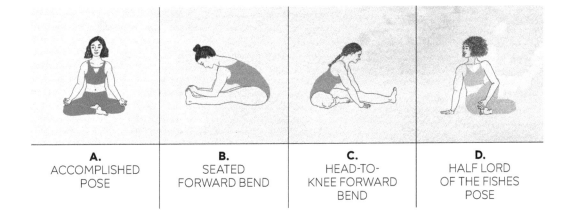

| **A.** ACCOMPLISHED POSE | **B.** SEATED FORWARD BEND | **C.** HEAD-TO-KNEE FORWARD BEND | **D.** HALF LORD OF THE FISHES POSE |

G. Anjaneyasana (Low Lunge, page 34)

H. Kapotasana (Pigeon Pose, page 40)

I. Malasana (Garland Pose, page 39)

J. Ardha Bhujangasana (Low Cobra Pose, page 61)

K. Bhujangasana (Cobra Pose, page 55)

L. Adho Mukha Svanasana (Downward-Facing Dog Pose, page 45)

M. Ashta Chandrasana (High Lunge, page 47)

N. Virabhadrasana II (Warrior II Pose, page 48)

O. Utthita Trikonasana (Extended Triangle Pose, page 54)

P. Natarajasana (Dancer Pose, page 58)

Q. Baddha Konasana (Bound-Angle Pose, page 35)

R. Upavistha Konasana (Wide-Angle Pose, page 38)

S. Navasana (Boat Pose, page 46)

T. Savasana (Corpse Pose, page 93)

Instructions:

1. Come into **Accomplished Pose**.

2. Stretch your legs out into **Seated Forward Bend**.

3. Bend the right leg and come into **Head-to-Knee Forward Bend** on the right.

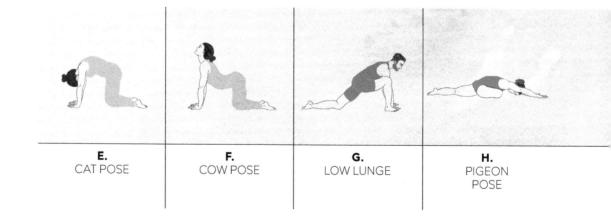

E.	F.	G.	H.
CAT POSE	COW POSE	LOW LUNGE	PIGEON POSE

4. Bend the left leg and come into **Half Lord of the Fishes Pose** on the right.

5. Stretch both legs out and come into **Head-to-Knee Forward Bend** on the left.

6. Move into **Half Lord of the Fishes Pose** on the left.

7. Come onto the hands and knees and move through **Cat** and **Cow Poses** for eight to ten repetitions, coordinating your movement with your breath. Inhale on the **Cow Pose** and exhale on the **Cat Pose**.

8. Step the right foot forward into **Low Lunge**.

9. Come straight into **Pigeon Pose** on the right.

10. Bring the right leg back and come into **Low Lunge** on the left.

11. Come straight into **Pigeon Pose** on the left.

12. Stand up and make your way into **Garland Pose**.

CONTINUED »

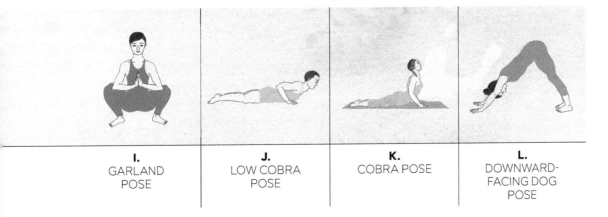

I.
GARLAND POSE

J.
LOW COBRA POSE

K.
COBRA POSE

L.
DOWNWARD-FACING DOG POSE

13. Come back to stand, then lie flat on your belly and move through three **Low Cobra Poses**.

14. Press up into **Cobra**.

15. Step back into **Downward-Facing Dog Pose**.

16. Step the right foot up into **High Lunge** on the right.

17. Shift into **Warrior II Pose** on the right.

18. Shift into **Extended Triangle Pose** on the right.

19. Come back through **Warrior II Pose** and into **Downward-Facing Dog Pose**.

20. Step the left foot into **High Lunge** on the left.

21. Shift into **Warrior II Pose** on the left.

22. Shift into **Extended Triangle Pose** on the left.

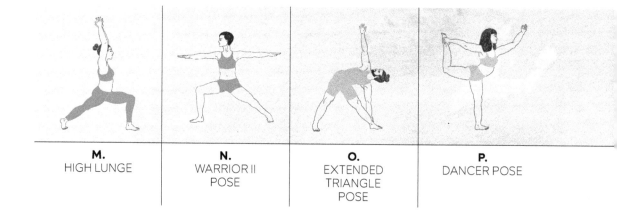

| **M.** HIGH LUNGE | **N.** WARRIOR II POSE | **O.** EXTENDED TRIANGLE POSE | **P.** DANCER POSE |

23. Make your way back into **Downward-Facing Dog Pose** and come up to stand.

24. Come into **Dancer Pose** on the right.

25. Come into **Dancer Pose** on the left.

26. Have a seat on the floor and move into **Bound-Angle Pose**.

27. Come into **Wide-Angle Pose**.

28. Come into **Boat Pose**.

29. Relax into **Savasana** for three to ten minutes.

TIP: Feel free to bend your knees in **Boat Pose** as a modification and use a strap in **Dancer Pose** if needed.

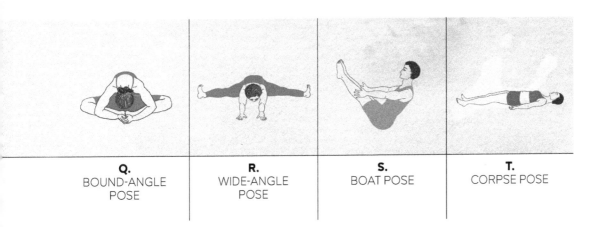

Q.
BOUND-ANGLE
POSE

R.
WIDE-ANGLE
POSE

S.
BOAT POSE

T.
CORPSE POSE

healing your inner self

Discover how to unblock and balance the entire chakra system by practicing yoga sequences that activate the full body.

Strength Building for the Whole Body

This yoga sequence is a full-body workout that activates all the chakras. This is a great well-rounded practice if you want to work on strengthening your muscles as well.

Props: Mat, blanket, block

Precautions: Use caution or avoid this sequence if you have recently had a knee, hip, back, leg, or arm injury or suffer from chronic pain in this area.

Benefits:
- Activates all chakras
- Strengthens the entire body
- Energizing
- Cardiovascular workout

Poses:

A. Prone Savasana (Prone Corpse Pose, page 81)

B. Anahatasana (Melting Heart Pose, page 63)

C. Anjaneyasana (Low Lunge, page 34)

D. Tadasana (Mountain Pose, page 92)

E. Kumbhakasana (Plank Pose, page 82)

F. Chaturanga Dandasana (Four-Limbed Staff Pose, page 83)

G. Urdhva Mukha Svanasana (Upward-Facing Dog Pose, page 56)

CONTINUED »

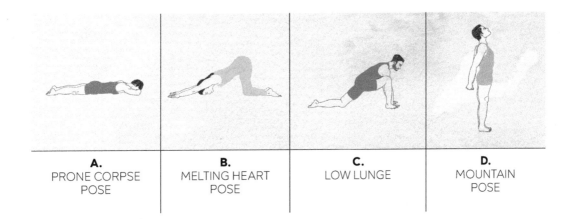

| **A.** PRONE CORPSE POSE | **B.** MELTING HEART POSE | **C.** LOW LUNGE | **D.** MOUNTAIN POSE |

H. Adho Mukha Svanasana (Downward-Facing Dog Pose, page 45)

I. Camatkarasana (Wild Thing, page 64)

J. Ashta Chandrasana (High Lunge, page 47)

K. Utthita Parsvakonasana (Extended Side-Angle Pose, page 97)

L. Ardha Matsyendrasana (Half Lord of the Fishes Pose, page 53)

M. Paschimottanasana (Seated Forward Bend, page 42)

N. Adho Mukha Vrksasana (Handstand, page 89)

O. Balasana (Child's Pose, page 80)

P. Savasana (Corpse Pose, page 93)

Instructions:

1. Come into **Prone Savasana**.

2. Press back into **Melting Heart Pose**.

3. Step the right leg into **Low Lunge** on the right.

4. Step the left leg into **Low Lunge** on the left.

5. Stand up into **Mountain Pose**.

6. Step back into **Plank Pose**.

7. Move into **Four-Limbed Staff Pose**.

8. Press up into **Upward-Facing Dog Pose**.

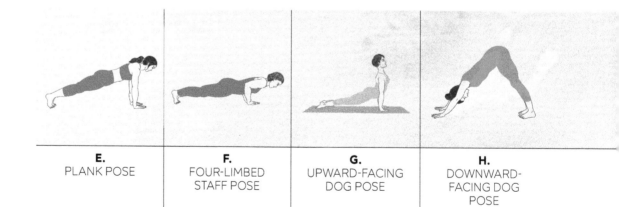

| **E.** PLANK POSE | **F.** FOUR-LIMBED STAFF POSE | **G.** UPWARD-FACING DOG POSE | **H.** DOWNWARD-FACING DOG POSE |

9. Press back into **Downward-Facing Dog Pose**.

10. Raise the right leg up behind you and step back into **Wild Thing** on the right.

11. Move back through **Downward-Facing Dog Pose**.

12. Step the right leg forward into **High Lunge** on the right side.

13. Shift into **Extended Side-Angle Pose** on the right side.

14. Come back through **High Lunge** and through **Downward-Facing Dog Pose**.

15. Raise the left leg up behind you and step into **Wild Thing** on the left.

16. Come back through **Downward-Facing Dog Pose**.

17. Step the left foot forward into **High Lunge** on the left.

18. Shift straight into **Extended Side-Angle Pose** on the left.

CONTINUED ››

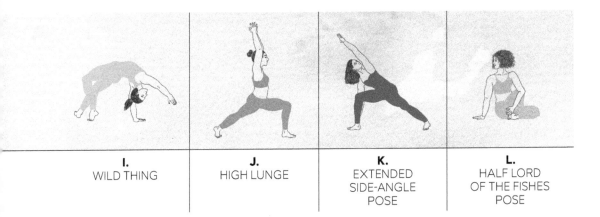

| **I.** WILD THING | **J.** HIGH LUNGE | **K.** EXTENDED SIDE-ANGLE POSE | **L.** HALF LORD OF THE FISHES POSE |

19. Come back through **High Lunge** and through **Downward-Facing Dog Pose**.

20. Come to sit.

21. Come into **Half Lord of the Fishes** on the right.

22. Repeat on the left.

23. Move into **Seated Forward Bend**.

24. Move to the wall and come into **Handstand** at the wall.

25. Come straight down and rest in **Child's Pose**.

26. Make your way into **Savasana** and hold for three to ten minutes.

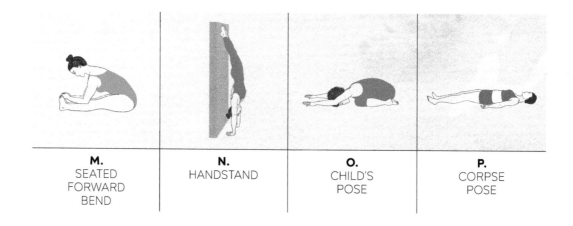

| **M.** SEATED FORWARD BEND | **N.** HANDSTAND | **O.** CHILD'S POSE | **P.** CORPSE POSE |

Energizing the Full Body

This is another sequence that activates the entire chakra system and is a full-body yoga routine. You can practice this routine if you are in need of an energy boost, as the poses are very uplifting and energizing.

Props: Mat, blanket, block

Precautions: Use caution or avoid this sequence if you have recently had a knee, hip, back, leg, or arm injury or suffer from chronic pain in any of these areas.

Benefits:
- Activates all chakras
- Energizes the body and mind
- Empowering
- Uplifting

Poses:

A. Salamba Matsyasana (Supported Fish Pose, page 74)

B. Sukhasana (Easy Pose, page 70)

C. Neck Rolls in Sukhasana: Easy Pose (page 72)

D. Assisted Neck Stretches in Sukhasana: Easy Pose (page 70)

E. Sukhasana with Jalandhara Bandha (Easy Pose with Chin Lock, page 73)

F. Balasana (Child's Pose, page 80)

CONTINUED »

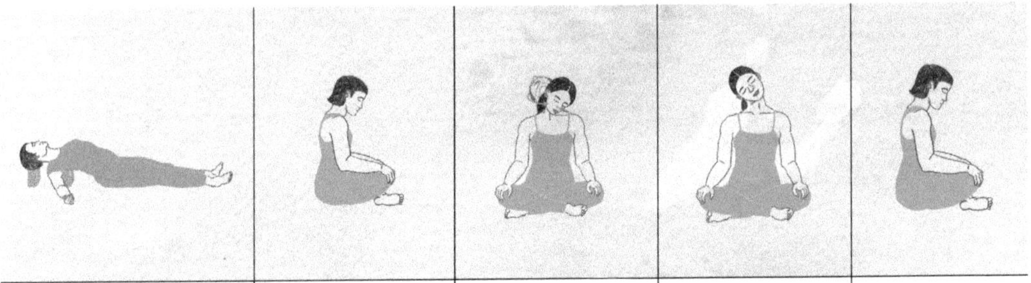

A. SUPPORTED FISH POSE	B. EASY POSE	C. EASY POSE	D. EASY POSE	E. EASY POSE WITH CHIN LOCK

G. Anahatasana (Melting Heart Pose, page 63)

H. Marjaryasana (Cat Pose, page 51)

I. Bitilasana (Cow Pose, page 52)

J. Ardha Bhujangasana (Low Cobra Pose, page 61)

K. Bhujangasana (Cobra Pose, page 55)

L. Tadasana (Mountain Pose, page 60)

M. Kumbhakasana (Plank Pose, page 82)

N. Chaturanga Dandasana (Four-Limbed Staff Pose, page 83)

O. Urdhva Mukha Svanasana (Upward-Facing Dog Pose, page 56)

P. Adho Mukha Svanasana (Downward-Facing Dog Pose, page 45)

Q. Ustrasana (Camel Pose, page 66)

R. Setu Bandha Sarvangasana (Bridge Pose, page 44)

S. Urdhva Dhanurasana (Upward-Facing Bow Pose, page 67)

T. Ardha Matsyendrasana (Half Lord of the Fishes Pose, page 53)

U. Savasana (Corpse Pose, page 93)

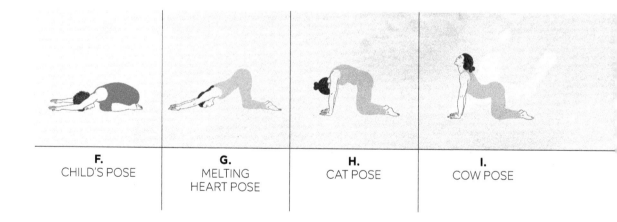

| **F.** CHILD'S POSE | **G.** MELTING HEART POSE | **H.** CAT POSE | **I.** COW POSE |

Instructions:

1. Arrange your props to come into **Supported Fish Pose** and relax there for one to three minutes.

2. Come up to sit in **Easy Pose** and move through your **Neck Rolls**.

3. Remain in **Easy Pose** and move into your **Assisted Neck Stretches**.

4. Bring the head back to center and come into **Easy Pose with Chin Lock**.

5. Come onto the hands and knees and into **Child's Pose**.

6. Come up into **Melting Heart Pose**.

7. Come onto the hands and knees and move through **Cat** and **Cow Poses** for eight to ten repetitions, coordinating your movement with your breath. Inhale on the **Cow Pose** and exhale on the **Cat Pose**.

8. Lie flat on your belly and lift up into **Low Cobra Pose** three times.

CONTINUED »

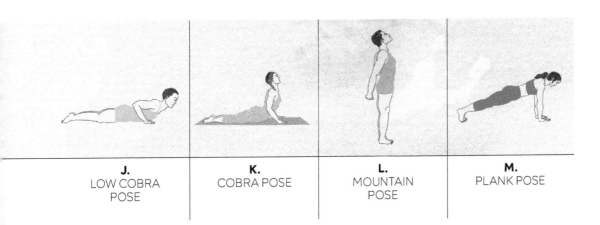

| **J.** LOW COBRA POSE | **K.** COBRA POSE | **L.** MOUNTAIN POSE | **M.** PLANK POSE |

9. Press up into **Cobra Pose**.

10. Stand up into **Mountain Pose**.

11. Step back into **Plank Pose**.

12. Move through **Four-Limbed Staff Pose** and straight into **Upward-Facing Dog Pose**.

13. Press back into **Downward-Facing Dog Pose**.

14. Come to your knees and move into **Camel Pose**.

15. Sit back into **Child's Pose**.

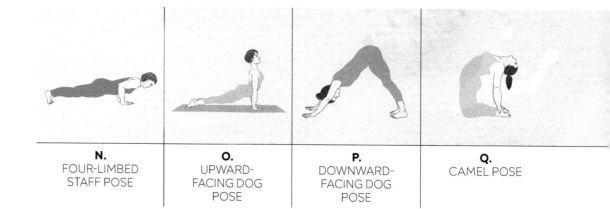

| N. FOUR-LIMBED STAFF POSE | O. UPWARD-FACING DOG POSE | P. DOWNWARD-FACING DOG POSE | Q. CAMEL POSE |

16. Lie flat on your back and move into **Bridge Pose**.

17. Press up into **Upward-Facing Bow Pose** two or three times.

18. Come into **Half Lord of the Fishes Pose** on the right.

19. Come into **Half Lord of the Fishes Pose** on the left.

20. Lie flat on your back, bend the knees, and hug both legs in toward the chest for three to five deep breaths.

21. Come into **Savasana** and rest there for three to ten minutes.

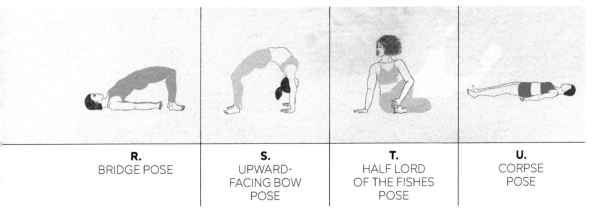

| **R.** BRIDGE POSE | **S.** UPWARD-FACING BOW POSE | **T.** HALF LORD OF THE FISHES POSE | **U.** CORPSE POSE |

Calming and Relaxing the Mind and Body

As opposed to the previous two sequences in this chapter, this full-body routine is restorative and calming. If you are feeling anxious or stressed, this is a great routine to practice.

Props: Mat, blanket, block

Precautions: Use caution or avoid this sequence if you have recently had a knee, hip, back, leg, or arm injury or suffer from chronic pain in any of these areas.

Benefits:
- Balances and relaxes the full chakra system
- Relaxes the body and mind

Poses:

A. Balasana (Child's Pose, page 80)

B. Anahatasana (Melting Heart Pose, page 63)

C. Ardha Bhujangasana (Low Cobra Pose, page 61)

D. Salamba Bhujangasana (Sphinx Pose, page 62)

E. Anjaneyasana (Low Lunge, page 34)

F. Kapotasana (Pigeon Pose, page 40)

G. Ardha Matsyendrasana (Half Lord of the Fishes Pose, page 53)

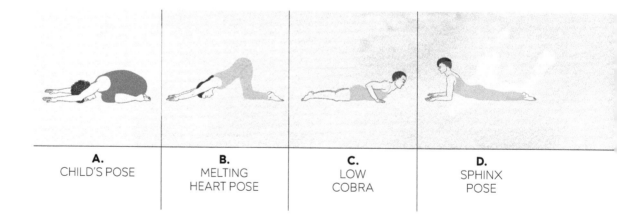

| **A.** CHILD'S POSE | **B.** MELTING HEART POSE | **C.** LOW COBRA | **D.** SPHINX POSE |

H. Paschimottanasana (Seated Forward Bend, page 42)

I. Janu Sirsasana (Head-to-Knee Forward Bend, page 43)

J. Baddha Konasana (Bound-Angle Pose, page 35)

K. Upavistha Konasana (Wide-Angle Pose, page 38)

L. Ananda Balasana (Happy Baby Pose, page 36)

M. Savasana (Corpse Pose, page 93)

Instructions:

1. Come onto your hands and knees and move into **Child's Pose**.

2. Come into **Melting Heart Pose**.

3. Lie flat on your belly and come into **Low Cobra Pose** three times.

4. Press up into **Sphinx Pose**.

5. Sit back into **Child's Pose**.

6. Come up onto your hands and knees and step the right foot forward into **Low Lunge** on the right side.

CONTINUED ››

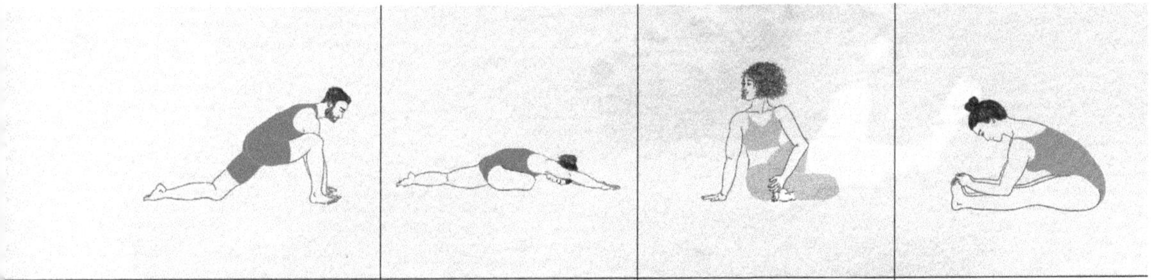

E. LOW LUNGE	**F.** PIGEON POSE	**G.** HALF LORD OF THE FISHES POSE	**H.** SEATED FORWARD BEND

7. Move straight into **Pigeon Pose** on the right side.

8. Come out of **Pigeon Pose** and move into **Half Lord of the Fishes Pose** on the right side.

9. Come out of **Half Lord of the Fishes Pose** and move into **Pigeon Pose** on the left side.

10. Come out of **Pigeon Pose** and move into **Half Lord of the Fishes Pose** on the left side.

11. Come back onto your hands and knees and step the left foot forward into **Low Lunge** on the left side.

12. Come to sit and move into **Seated Forward Bend**.

13. Move into **Head-to-Knee Forward Bend** on the right.

14. Move into **Head-to-Knee Forward Bend** on the left.

15. Come into **Bound-Angle Pose**.

16. Come into **Wide-Angle Pose**.

17. Lie flat on your back, bend your knees, and hug the legs in toward the chest. Hold for three to five deep breaths.

18. Move into **Happy Baby Pose**.

19. Straighten the legs out into **Savasana** and relax there for three to five minutes.

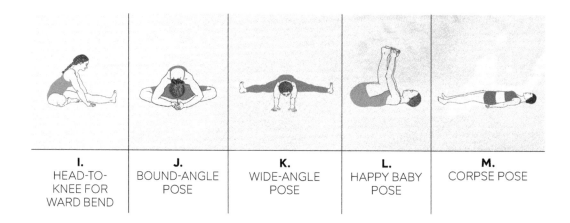

| **I.** HEAD-TO-KNEE FOR WARD BEND | **J.** BOUND-ANGLE POSE | **K.** WIDE-ANGLE POSE | **L.** HAPPY BABY POSE | **M.** CORPSE POSE |

Keeping the Full Body Grounded and Centered

As with the previous routine, this one is relaxing, but it is more grounding and centering. If you are suffering from anxiety or a lot of stress, this will help slow your heart rate and bring you back to reality.

Props: Mat, blanket, block

Precautions: Use caution or avoid this sequence if you have recently had a knee, hip, back, leg, or arm injury or suffer from chronic pain in any of these areas.

Benefits:
- Calming for the body and mind
- Grounding and centering
- Relaxing
- A full-body yoga routine

Poses:

A. Marjaryasana (Cat Pose, page 51)

B. Bitilasana (Cow Pose, page 52)

C. Adho Mukha Svanasana (Downward-Facing Dog Pose, page 45)

D. Anjaneyasana (Low Lunge, page 34)

E. Ashta Chandrasana (High Lunge, page 47)

F. Uttanasana (Standing Forward Bend, page 76)

G. Tadasana (Mountain Pose, page 60)

CONTINUED »

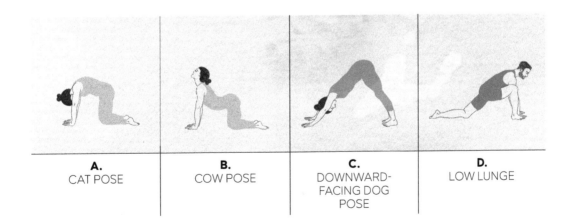

A. CAT POSE	**B.** COW POSE	**C.** DOWNWARD-FACING DOG POSE	**D.** LOW LUNGE

H. Utthita Trikonasana (Extended Triangle Pose, page 54)

I. Prasarita Padottanasana I (Wide-Legged Forward Bend, page 37)

J. Utkata Konasana (Goddess Pose, page 49)

K. Baddha Konasana Variation (Butterfly Pose, page 85)

L. Viparita Karani (Legs Up the Wall Pose, page 84)

M. Prone Savasana (Prone Corpse Pose, page 81)

Instructions:

1. Come onto the hands and knees and move through **Cat** and **Cow Poses** for eight to ten repetitions, coordinating your movement with your breath. Inhale on the **Cow Pose** and exhale on the **Cat Pose**.

2. Come into **Downward-Facing Dog Pose**.

3. Step the right leg forward into **Low Lunge** on the right side.

4. Step back into **Downward-Facing Dog Pose**.

5. Step the left leg forward into **Low Lunge** on the left side.

6. Step back into **Downward-Facing Dog Pose**.

7. Step the right leg forward into **High Lunge** on the right side.

8. Step back into **Downward-Facing Dog Pose**.

9. Step the left leg forward into **High Lunge** on the left side.

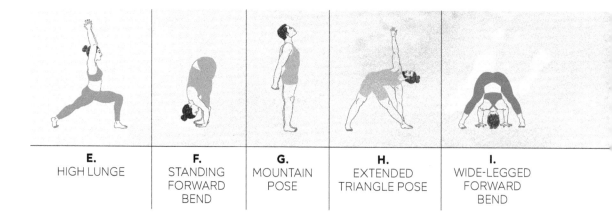

E. HIGH LUNGE	**F.** STANDING FORWARD BEND	**G.** MOUNTAIN POSE	**H.** EXTENDED TRIANGLE POSE	**I.** WIDE-LEGGED FORWARD BEND

10. Step back into **Downward-Facing Dog Pose**.

11. Raise the heels, bend the knees and look forward, then step the feet up, one foot at a time, into **Standing Forward Bend**.

12. Stand up into **Mountain Pose**.

13. Step the feet out wide and come into **Extended Triangle Pose** on the right side.

14. Come up to standing and move into **Wide-Legged Forward Bend**.

15. Come up to standing and move into **Extended Triangle Pose** on the left side.

16. Come up to standing and move into **Goddess Pose**.

17. Come to a seated position and move into **Butterfly Pose**.

18. Come to a wall and move into **Legs Up the Wall Pose**.

19. Move into **Prone Savasana** and remain there for three to eight minutes.

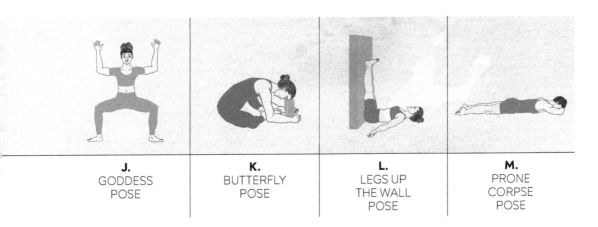

J.
GODDESS
POSE

K.
BUTTERFLY
POSE

L.
LEGS UP
THE WALL
POSE

M.
PRONE
CORPSE
POSE

INDEX

A

Adho Mukha Svanasana (Downward-Facing Dog Pose), 45
Adho Mukha Vrksasana (Handstand), 89–90
Anahatasana (Melting Heart Pose), 63
Ananda Balasana (Happy Baby Pose), 36
Anjaneyasana (Low Lunge), 34
Anjaneyasana Variation (Crescent Lunge with Arms Up), 95
Ardha Bhujangasana (Low Cobra Pose), 61
Ardha Chandrasana (Half-Moon Pose), 98
Ardha Matsyendrasana (Half Lord of the Fishes Pose), 53
Aromatherapy, 19
Asana practice, 4
Ashta Chandrasana (High Lunge), 47
Ashtangasana (Knees, Chest, Chin Pose), 75

B

Baddha Konasana (Bound-Angle Pose), 35
Baddha Konasana Variation (Butterfly Pose), 85–86
Balance, 4, 7–8, 11
Balasana (Child's Pose), 80
Bandhas (locks), 25–26
Bhujangasana (Cobra Pose), 55
Bitilasana (Cow Pose), 51
Blockages, 3, 7, 17–18. *See also Granthis* (knots)
Body, listening to, 22–23
Body scanning, 16, 18
Breath, 24–25

C

Camatkarasana (Wild Thing), 64
Chakras, 3. *See also specific*
    balancing, 21
    blocked, 7–8, 17–18
    major, 10–14
    minor, 15
    unblocking, 18–19
Chaturanga Dandasana (Four-Limbed Staff Pose), 83
Clothing, 28
Commitment, 6
Compassion, 6, 28
Crown chakra, 14, 91
    Anjaneyasana Variation (Crescent Lunge with Arms Up), 95
    Ardha Chandrasana (Half-Moon Pose), 98
    Salamba Sirsasana (Supported Headstand), 99–100
    Savasana (Corpse Pose), 93
    Tadasana (Mountain Pose), 92
    Utthita Parsvakonasana (Extended Side-Angle Pose), 97
    Vasisthasana (Side Plank Pose), 96
    Vrksasana (Tree Pose), 94
Crystals, 19

D

Dance, 27
Dhanurasana (Bow Pose), 57

E

"Edge," finding your, 24
Emotions, 26
Energy, 3, 7, 11, 24

F

Feelings, 26

G

Goal setting, 22
Gomukhasana (Cow Face Pose), 87–88
Granthis (knots), 25

H

Halasana (Plow Pose), 77
Heart chakra, 13, 59
    Anahatasana (Melting Heart Pose), 63
    Ardha Bhujangasana (Low Cobra Pose), 61
    Camatkarasana (Wild Thing), 64
    Matsyasana (Fish Pose), 65
    Salamba Bhujangasana (Sphinx/Supported
      Cobra Pose), 62
    Tadasana (Mountain Pose), 60
    Urdhva Dhanurasana (Upward-Facinig
      Bow/Wheel Pose), 67–68
    Ustrasana (Camel Pose), 66

I

Imbalances, 3

J

Jalandhara Bandha, 25
Janu Sirsasana (Head-to-Knee Forward Bend), 43

K

Kapotasana (Pigeon Pose), 40
Kumbhakasana (Plank Pose), 82

M

Maha Bandha, 25
Malasana (Garland Pose), 39
Marjaryasana (Cat Pose), 52
Mats, 22, 28
Matsyasana (Fish Pose), 65
Meditation, 18
Mind-body connection, 8
Mula Bandha, 25

N

Natarajasana (Dancer Pose), 58
Natya, 27
Navasana (Boat Pose), 46
Nritta, 27
Nritya, 27

P

Pain, 23
Paschimottanasana (Seated Forward Bend), 42
Poses, 5, 23–24. *See also specific*
Prana, 3, 7, 11, 16, 24, 27
Prasarita Padottanasana I (Wide-Legged
    Forward Bend), 37
Props, 28

R

Reiki, 19
Root chakra, 11, 32
    Ananda Balasana (Happy Baby Pose), 36
    Anjaneyasana (Low Lunge), 34
    Baddha Konasana (Bound-Angle Pose), 35
    Kapotasana (Pigeon Pose), 40
    Malasana (Garland Pose), 39
    Prasarita Padottanasana I (Wide-Legged
      Forward Bend), 37

Root chakra (*Continued*)
  Siddhasana (Accomplished Pose), 33
  Upavistha Konasana (Wide-Angle Pose), 38

S

Sacral chakra, 12, 41
  Adho Mukha Svanasana (Downward-Facing
    Dog Pose), 45
  Ashta Chandrasana (High Lunge), 47
  Janu Sirsasana (Head-to-Knee
    Forward Bend), 43
  Navasana (Boat Pose), 46
  Paschimottanasana (Seated Forward Bend), 42
  Setu Bandha Sarvangasana (Bridge Pose), 44
  Utkata Konasana (Goddess Pose), 49
  Virabhadrasana II (Warrior II Pose), 48
Salamba Bhujangasana (Sphinx/Supported
    Cobra Pose), 62
Salamba Matsyasana (Supported Fish Pose), 74
Salamba Sarvangasana (Supported Shoulder
    Stand), 78
Salamba Sirsasana (Supported
    Headstand), 99–100
Savasana (Corpse Pose), 16, 93
  prone, 81
Setu Bandha Sarvangasana (Bridge Pose), 44
Siddhasana (Accomplished Pose), 33
Solar plexus chakra, 12, 50
  Ardha Matsyendrasana (Half Lord of the
    Fishes Pose), 53
  Bhujangasana (Cobra Pose), 55
  Bitilasana (Cow Pose), 52
  Dhanurasana (Bow Pose), 57
  Marjaryasana (Cat Pose), 51
  Natarajasana (Dancer Pose), 58
  Urdhva Mukha Svanasana
    (Upward-Facing Dog Pose), 56

Utthita Trikonasana
    (Extended Triangle Pose), 54
Sukhasana (Easy Pose)
  assisted neck stretches in, 70–71
  with Jalandhara Bandha (Chin Lock), 73
  neck rolls in, 72

T

Tadasana (Mountain Pose), 60, 92
Third-eye chakra, 14, 79
  Adho Mukha Vrksasana (Handstand), 89–90
  Baddha Konasana Variation
    (Butterfly Pose), 85–86
  Balasana (Child's Pose), 80
  Chaturanga Dandasana
    (Four-Limbed Staff Pose), 83
  Gomukhasana (Cow Face Pose), 87–88
  Kumbhakasana (Plank Pose), 82
  Prone Savasana (Prone Corpse Pose), 81
  Viparita Karani (Legs Up the Wall Pose), 84
Throat chakra, 13, 69
  Ashtangasana (Knees, Chest, Chin Pose), 75
  Halasana (Plow Pose), 77
  Salamba Matsyasana (Supported
    Fish Pose), 74
  Salamba Sarvangasana (Supported Shoulder
    Stand), 78
  Sukhasana (Easy Pose) with assisted neck
    stretches, 70–71
  Sukhasana (Easy Pose) with Jalandhara
    Bandha (Chin Lock), 73
  Sukhasana (Easy Pose) with neck rolls, 72
  Uttanasana (Standing Forward Bend), 76

U

Uddiyana Bandha, 25
Upavistha Konasana (Wide-Angle Pose), 38

Urdhva Dhanurasana (Upward-Facinig
    Bow/Wheel Pose), 67–68
Urdhva Mukha Svanasana (Upward-Facing
    Dog Pose), 56
Ustrasana (Camel Pose), 66
Utkata Konasana (Goddess Pose), 49
Uttanasana (Standing Forward Bend), 76
Utthita Parsvakonasana (Extended
    Side-Angle Pose), 97
Utthita Trikonasana (Extended
    Triangle Pose), 54

V

Vasisthasana (Side Plank Pose), 96
Viparita Karani (Legs Up the
    Wall Pose), 84
Virabhadrasana II (Warrior II Pose), 48
Vrksasana (Tree Pose), 94

Y

Yoga
    creating a practice, 21–23
    healing power of, 4–5
    preparing for practice, 28
Yoga sequences
    activating and grounding the
        midsection, 102–104
    building a strong foundation, 111–115
    calming and relaxing the mind and
        body, 126–128
    drawing attention and focus to the upper
        chakras, 105–107
    energizing the full body, 121–125
    keeping the full body grounded and
        centered, 129–131
    paying attention to the extremities, 108–110
    strength building for the whole body, 117–120

ACKNOWLEDGMENTS

Writing this book has been a grueling and rewarding process, and I have a great amount of gratitude for all the individuals who helped me along the way. First, I am very grateful to Callisto Media for allowing me this opportunity to share my knowledge of yoga with a wider audience through this book. I would like to thank Sean Newcott for her patience and understanding throughout the writing process, as well as the many others involved. Gratitude also goes to my yoga mentors, specifically Dani Zuccheri, for helping shape my yoga practice and teaching philosophy. I would like to thank my parents, Lisa and Joe, for their lifetime of love and support. Finally, thanks to my partner in life, Barry, who has to put up with me on a daily basis, and for that, I am forever grateful.

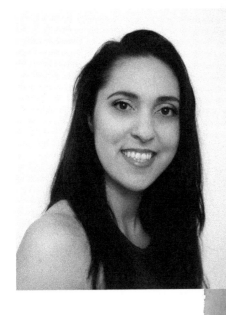

ABOUT THE AUTHOR

Christina D'Arrigo is a 500-hour-trained yoga teacher and former dancer/choreographer from New York City. As a former attendee of the *Fame* school in New York City, Christina received her specialized high school diploma in dance and then went on to study dance further in Los Angeles and London, where she received her bachelor's and master's degrees in dance and choreography. Upon her return to New York City, she completed her 500-hour yoga teacher training and began teaching yoga in live classes and online for thousands of people all over the world via the YouTube channel Yoga With Christina – ChriskaYoga and various other platforms.

Printed in the USA
CPSIA information can be obtained
at www.ICGtesting.com
CBHW082105210224
4500CB00011B/19